I0772559

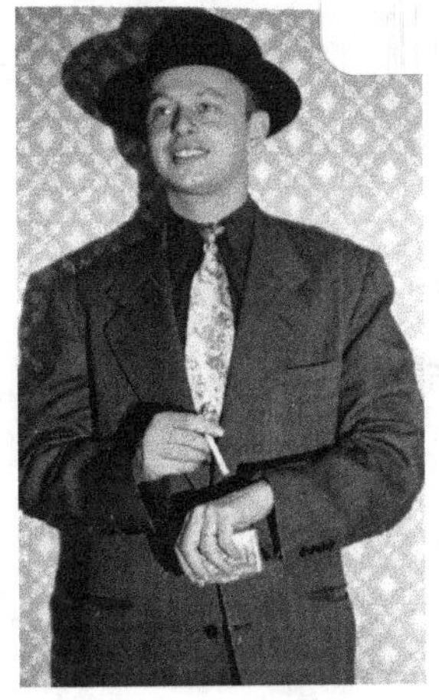

Benson Meth (c.1946)

EVERY DAY IS A GIFT

Surviving Cancer
and
Making Peace with the Past:
A Memoir
of
Love, Duty, and Friendship
Laughter, Tears, and Closure

by

DAVID L. METH

Writers' Productions
P.O. Box 630
Westport, CT 06881
DavidMeth.com

Copyright ©2018 by David L. Meth
All rights reserved.

ISBN: 9781983141768

No portion of this work may be copied, revised, derived, adapted, altered, transmitted, translated, published, or used in any way or in any language, including digital transmission in computer codes or languages from any device to another, online or wireless, without prior written permission from the author.

First Edition ©2018
Printed in the United States of America

This book is dedicated to my father who told me
"Every day is a gift."
And to my wife, Tomoko,
Whose love and perseverance has made it so.

• • •

My love also goes out to my friend Zev.
Your spirit is always with us.

• • •

And to my friends Danny and Roy …
Without you I would never have made it
during those early years.

Table of Contents

CHAPTER ONE

The Decision and My Next Cocktail

The thought of cancer makes you wince. It takes your breath away. It didn't hit me until I sat down in front of a computer to provide information at the local Red Cross in order to give blood. Halfway into the questions, I said that I had been diagnosed with the early stages of prostate cancer and the attendant paused. The pleasant smile drained from her face and she told me that her father was in the early stages of prostate cancer, too. Unfortunately, I would be unable to donate blood. I was disqualified. It had never occurred to me that I would be unfit as I entered the Red Cross storefront that morning, so I went to the lobby to wait for my wife, who was also giving blood, and reconsidered my life.

According to a stranger, even though I was in good health and fit otherwise, perfect health now had a new definition, and I didn't meet the requirements. Up to that moment, although I understood the implications of prostate cancer, it did not register until someone I was meeting for the first time looked me in the eye and told me I am not the person I thought I was when I walked in, and I had to take a breath.

But I was aware of cancer and its long reach. My father died from prostate cancer that, by the time he was diagnosed with it, had spread throughout his body. He was a guy who never liked to go to the doctor; so 30 years before my diagnosis, I watched him go from walking, to walking with a cane, to balancing himself on crutches, steadying himself with a walker, doing wheelies in a wheelchair, to a hospice, to a nursing home, to the hospital, and finally to the funeral home. That was in 1982, just shy of his 60th birthday; and although medical science and technology have improved dramatically since then, my memories had remained fixed on the two years leading up to his death and how it affected my whole family then and years later.

Now, I have come to understand that memories build up in layers from single events, to events that overlap and lead into each other, to narrative threads that color your thoughts and inform your decisions for years to come. The past helps to identify who you are compared to who you think you are. Consciously or subconsciously, serious illness, especially cancer, becomes an interpretation of life because someone who dies of cancer does not pleasantly "pass on" as many people like to eulogize. Cancer is brutal and punishing, and death takes away some of the life from the people who survive the patient. But you die, too, if only in small increments for a moment at a time. How long that moment lasts is up to you. It is only after reconciliation with death and peace among the living that the person who dies passes on. So, at the age of 64, 31 years after my father's death, I knew what could be and I was compelled to look back at who I was in order to discover who I had become.

• • •

Since my father's death, I was diligent about my health and had annual checkups. Twice a year for ten years leading up to my diagnosis, my urologist asked me to drop my pants, as he put on surgical gloves and thrilled me with questions about what I had for dinner or where I went on my last vacation, while his fingers went to a place that only he could visit. I monitored my PSA (prostate-specific antigen) numbers as they went up very slowly until the level of elevation went beyond 4.0 and he suggested that I should have a biopsy. That was a week before a massive flood of news, starting with an article in the New York Times Magazine on Oct. 9, 2011, that reported the PSA was unnecessary at best and, at worst, may convince you to do procedures that will change your life forever. Either way, cancer changes your life. Now what?

There was little doubt in my mind, or my wife's, that I should at least go for the preliminary tests in order to make a decision. The biopsy was in-office, quick and painless, but it came back with four random spots of cancer in my prostate gland. "Random" is an important word because it meant only what was found. There could be more. As confirmed by other articles, however: So what? Prostate cancer may remain in your body and never affect you. My Gleason score with an average of 4 meant that the cancer was not aggressive. That was good. Just walk away. My doctor was not convinced and suggested further examination to be certain. Nothing to be concerned about, but "better safe than sorry," as my father used to say, but never set as an example. Good news, all in all. So I agreed to go for my first CAT scan and faced the original Donut Drive-through: a big white plastic circle with a gurney that moves you back and forth through the hole in the center that shoots you up with radiation while a robotic voice suggests that you are in good hands, in the 2001 Space Odyssey sense.

First the preparation: Which arm would you like to use for the contrast liquid? It may make you a bit warm and leave a funny taste in your mouth. You may have the urge to urinate, although you won't actually urinate, but get used to the feeling. These are normal side effects. You'll also be dehydrated. Any questions? Yes, uh, could you … Please put on the gown and lie on your back. Everybody out. No, not you. What am I, a mutant? Well, not yet, but I was the only one left unprotected. Then a cute fat yellow face that looks like a balloon about to explode tells you in bold terms to hold your breath. Wait … One … Two … Three … Four … Take a deep breath. Now hold. Next a little round green face with an open mouth tells you to breathe again. Hold your breath. Breathe. Hold your breath. Breathe. There is no end to the cute surprises. Between the balloon faces is a digital read-out of clear, bright yellow numbers that start in the hundreds and I assume is the price for each scan per second. First pass: 136.43—Okay. Reasonable for cancer scanning. Besides, I gotta do it. Next read-out: 545.72—That went up quickly. There goes any thoughts of a weekend get away. Third read-out: 682.15. Pardon me, am I in network? What's my deductible? I think I'll skip the third pass. Please see the collections desk up front. CAT scan: clean. Following that, I had a bone scan. The good news: no problem. The real news: See you back next year for the rest of your life—according to the technician who didn't know the reason for my bone scan. Apparently that was the reaction for people with bone problems. Luckily, that scan came back negative. I was clean again. No need to return. I think. What did he know, anyway?

Now I had to put this all together and make a decision: Let these low grade, early stage indications of cancer remain untreated because prostate cancer grows very slowly and I may never be affected by it according to recent studies, or ... Should I consider treatment because of the personal history that I now shared with my father. Of course, this condition did not reveal itself suddenly one morning or catch me by surprise. I had an enlarged prostate gland that kept me up and in the bathroom six to eight times a night and made me wander around like a zombie with my hands outstretched, groping for balance during the day until I managed to squeeze in a nap or infused myself with coffee that, by the way, does not go well with plans to take a nap. So I had a TURP (transurethral resection of the prostate), surgery to hollow out my prostate gland and wore a catheter for two weeks which was ... and please take this in the unique way it provides relief ... Wonnnderful! I did not have to get up at all during the night to go to the bathroom.

As per doctor's advisory for one of the side effects that rarely happens and that I shouldn't worry about, I developed a blood clot in my urinary tract for one endless Sunday night of shivering, shaking, and more pain than I ever want to experience again in my life: a small reward in what would be my ongoing efforts to end my hourly journeys to the bathroom every night for the previous ten sleepless years. Of course, this was only one of the possible side effects. Oh, yes. Sleep deprivation—the words that doctors cannot find in their textbooks unless it applied to their residencies, and are omitted in brochures describing procedures and side effects. Let me spell it out for the medical professionals reading this book: S-L-E-E-P D-E-P-R-I-V-A-T-I-O-N!

I asked my urologist if I could put my decision off to consider what treatment to do, or if at all, and he agreed that I could. Great. For a month. A month? How about a year? It would take me at least that long to read and digest all the information that was flooding the media and the Internet against using the PSA as a measure for prostate cancer treatment. I could postpone or not even do the treatment, he answered; but if the cancer spreads to the bone or any other place in my body, I would have a much different problem. Yes, Dad, you proved that. The doctor gave me very specific information about my options, and my wife and I did more research to try and understand my situation and the ramifications of not taking action, as well as pursuing treatment. It didn't any get easier, as I learned that the most serious problems are not due to the cancer of the prostate gland, but that the choices of procedures produced side effects that were intrusive and disturbing physically and emotionally, even humiliating. This was going to be fun: Choose between Column A: incontinence; Column B: impotence, or all of the above, and for those who place their order immediately: The Super Special—Insomnia.

My urologist suggested that I see the head of Radiation Oncology at my local hospital that had a dedicated Cancer Center, and I could always get a second, or other opinions from any hospital or doctors of my choice. This was already too much to think about. But it could not be delayed, because to avoid it would have quite foreseeable consequences. So, with the ten-year record of my rising PSA, the biopsy, the Gleason score, the CAT scan and bone scan, I went to my local hospital to see the head of Radiation Oncology, a very nice man about my age with an excellent sense of humor. I had already lived 5 years longer than my father, thanks to my wife's excellent cooking and the local gym where I exercised at least 3-4 days a week, and go to 7 days a week to sit in the steam or sauna with long-time friends and talk politics, news, sports, and the pleasures of creeping into our 50s, 60s, and beyond. What we were all gradually realizing was that, together, we were a great source of information about health, nutrition, and various ailments and infirmities that come with aging. Naturally, up for discussion were medical professionals, health insurance, and the one rule you must live by: to stay healthy you must eat nutritious food, exercise your mind as well as your body, and maintain long-term friendships with good people. Oh, and have a deeply appreciative, even ironic sense of humor, because laughter is as much a cure for any illness as medication: It fits together the puzzle pieces of your past in ways that you could not have envisioned before. It also tests your tolerance of irony with a sprinkling of sarcasm that is passed on to the survivors, as it was from my father to me at the most unlikely moments.

• • •

One day, when I was visiting him at the hospital, I went down to fill a couple of pitchers with ice, the only drink he could have and, basically, not much more for lunch or dinner, except for Jell-O and the pleasant smiles of the people who served him. There was a lot going on. A very recent acquaintance of my father's, a short, elderly grandmother was looking for her husband. He was senile and had to be watched closely as he set off one alarm after another walking into areas where he shouldn't be. Several nurses dashed out of the emergency exit and came back with an elderly man wearing a hat, a white shirt and tie, and dressed in his underwear, He also had his belongings under his arm. I told my father about the adventure and he sneered: "It's probably one of the doctors." In spite of my father's suffering, he still had the ability to make me laugh. And I loved him for it.

CHAPTER TWO

In My Doctor's Hands

From my father's experience to mine, I knew what to expect in my new doctor's hands. Well, I thought I knew based on prior years of visits to the medical professionals until he asked me to bend over and spread my legs. He then proceeded to shove his finger up to my scalp through my rectum to examine my prostate gland. "Prostate is smooth," he said with great clinical indifference. Somebody help me straighten up, thank you. He hosed his arm down, and with a smile asked me to get dressed and come into his office. Alone? Oh, no you don't. I brought my wife. If anyone thinks he can, or should, consider cancer and its treatment on his own: Reconsider. You need the comfort and assurance of someone close to you, family or friend, to listen, take notes, ask questions and discuss everything before, during, and after you decide what you are going to do because it is overwhelming. You need someone special by your side.

My Doctor of Expert Radiation next directed our attention to a large laminated poster of the male body and went through every detail of the prostate gland and the options to treat prostate cancer. Questions started to flood my mind: Should I get another opinion? Should I take a chance and wait and see how this very slow cancer develops? Should I opt for immediate treatment while my insurance will cover the costs, at least on paper? Yes, you have to consider expenses that are enormous because, as the doctor said, "It will eat up your deductible like an hors d'oeuvre." But I had to ask him: "Shouldn't I go to a world renowned cancer care center?"

He didn't take offense and replied, "Of course, you can always expect great care at a famous hospital. (He was being kind, as I have had experiences quite contrary to the reputation of certain "world renowned" hospitals.) However, you will be just another number, one more case for that day. It's impersonal. Here, you get a personal touch."

"Excuse me? You just shoved your fist up my rectum until you couldn't see your elbow." He tried his best not to laugh, but it didn't work. "I think I know what you mean by a personal touch." I looked at my wife and she put her head in her hands to disguise her effort not to laugh. "No need for me to go for a second opinion." My wife agreed. We all laughed, and the doctor brought over a 4"x4" black cube with small holes and numbers. He placed some very thin, 12" long pins that looked like needles next to it.

"This is where the seeds are going," he explained.

"Into the block?"

"Through the block."

"Oh, yeah? How exactly are you going to get this numeric game cube inside my body, and where did you have in mind to put it?"

He laughed.

This is funny?

"Will the corners protrude? Cables coming out to a computer?"

He stared at me in astonishment. "Are you serious?"

I smiled sarcastically. "Are you serious?"

"This is the guide."

The guide?

"You are not going anywhere near my internal organs with a 4"x4" cube. I'll go online and hire my own guide. Maybe we'll put together a medical safari."

"It's for your urologist to guide the seed implementation."

"You mean for those dozen or so curtain rods he's going to insert into my prostate gland in order to deposit the seeds? How about a Lego set and chopsticks? Straws to blow them through?"

"It stays outside your body."

Please, just put me out and tell me when it's over. Maybe in a year or two.

We asked about medication, follow-ups, and side effects. Everything. Well, almost everything. We never discussed the side effects of the side effects. What? Side effects mean side effects, right? No, not quite. We'll come to that later, as the journey continues from the basic information, to the details, to the questions, to **The Decision**. But first the choices:

1. External Beam: You go in every day at a time of your choice for 10 minutes or so, 5 days on, 2 days off for about 8 weeks. That means at least 30 minutes to an hour a day, door-to-door depending on where you are coming from. Although radiation comes from the outside and is highly focused on a minute, clear, predetermined spot, it still goes through other parts of your body. Nope. Maybe

I'm still haunted by my father's primitive treatments, but I don't want any other part of my body touched, irradiated, nuked, violated, or destroyed.

2. Surgery: Remove the prostate gland and re-attach everything. That would bring the PSA down to zero, but eliminate sex and other types of intense exercise for the rest of my life because something might separate or detach and cause other problems. Don't think so. Besides, that's a last resort. Even at 64, I was too young for that procedure.

3. Watchful Waiting: Sit it out and see what happens—not with my father's history.

4. Seed implants: One surgery, dozens of tiny pellets that would stay in my body and grow in intensity for 4 weeks and die over the following weeks up to about ten because of their radioactive half-life. I would also smolder in the dark as I peed with day-glow colors and shoot neon pellets during sex—no, that's been eliminated. Did I mention getting patted down at the airport because I am radioactive (if the TSA isn't distracted by the titanium in my hip—please, don't ask. Well, maybe in another chapter of this treatise on the thrill of survival). No one bothered to tell me that I wouldn't sleep more than 30-

60 minutes at a stretch at night for at least 4 months, while blindly holding a strainer in front of me in the dark to catch any renegade nuclear mini-missiles. Call HazMat. No trouble finding me. Look for the house that flashes on and off like a strobe light after midnight. Do I hear disco music?

I opted for the nuclear implants. Little did the pamphlets, the brochures, and the doctors have any idea beyond the boilerplate explanation of the side effects about how I, a human being, would actually be affected. The doctors should know, but they do not draw at least one obvious conclusion from the questions they ask: How often you do get up at night? Does your urine burn? How is the stream? Any blood? Catch any nuclear residue or set off any dirty bombs? No, they never think to ask how long you sleep before you get up again. When you get up 6 to 8 times a night, even if you get back to sleep, you're up. Soon, you can audition for a 1950's grade B horror flick as you walk around like Boris Karloff in The Mummy, because sleep deprivation is cumulative. You start dropping things. You make turns that are too narrow and bump into corners. You forget what you have to do and where you are. Have you seen my glasses? Where are my car keys? And … you drive? Okay, let's go shopping. Yes, you still have to go to work to earn a living. **SLEEP DEPRIVATION**: all the other side effects put together, including those directly related to the surgery and medications that, if you read the labels carefully, make having a root canal done without anesthesia and then being buried alive a most pleasant and desirable experience.

The next natural step was to read the warning on the labels of the medications that clearly emphasized what most people would **never** really experience. Oh, yeah? Well, why the disclaimer? Why the discount coupon for the local embalmer? Please be advised, these few side effects, though rare, might occur, so if they do, don't say you weren't warned: Constipation and diarrhea—at the same time? How exactly does that work? Dizziness, gas, headache and heartburn—okay, I get plenty of that when we get together with my mother for dinner every month and on holidays. Nausea—all the time: Try to digest the speeches given by politicians. Not on a full stomach, please.

Sore throat, stomach upset, clogged nose—it's called a virus. However, if these symptoms get worse, seek medical attention right away, especially if you have: severe rash, hives, itching, trouble breathing, tightness in the chest—a bee sting, allergies, **and** a heart attack? Swelling of the mouth, face, lips, or tongue—From what? I haven't been out of the county, no less the country. Cancel all public speaking engagements.

Bloody or black, tarry stools—What the fuck? Change in the amount of urine produced—okay, that's a given, given the surgery. Any other problems? Chest pain. Doesn't that precede a heart attack? Confusion—nailed me: I'm confused. Dark urine—bloody, dark urine? Again? Depression—You're succeeding. Fainting—I'm ready. Fast or irregular heartbeat—I'm experiencing that now. Fever, chills, or persistent sore throat—Anything else?

Hearing loss, mental or mood changes—lock me up in a padded room. Prone to violence—shall I turn myself in ahead of time to prevent harm to others? Numbness of an arm or leg, one-sided weakness—Why go on living? Red, swollen, blistered, or peeling skin—Are you out of your fucking mind? Ringing in the ears—to follow the headache I'm getting? Seizures—and this is a medication? Severe headache or dizziness …caused by … the seizures?

And this is the cure? Severe or persistent stomach pain or nausea—I can't take much more. Severe vomiting—That's one way to lose weight. Shortness of breath—I can barely breathe now. Sudden or unexplained weight gain—I just lost 15 pounds. Forget it. Swelling of hands, legs, or feet—Again? Just amputate them and carry me around in a basket. Unusual bruising or bleeding—From what? I'll never get out of bed after reading this. Unusual joint or muscle pain—at least the bleeding stopped. Unusual tiredness or weakness—Like reading this gives me strength, energy and confidence. Vision or speech changes—I'm already wearing bifocals and mumbling to people only I can see, as I teach my students and walk on the street alone. Vomit that looks like coffee grinds—Isn't that what you get at the supermarket? Yellowing of the skin or eyes—At least I can audition as a vampire and make a few million dollars in the movies to cover the out-of-network medical bills. But this is not a complete list of all side effects that may occur, in which case, please make sure your life insurance is up to date, create a new will and have a family member sign for power of attorney. Oh, don't forget to make funeral arrangements before you check in.

So I made my decision and the day was approaching. I had to prepare. Among the medications I had to take was the equivalent of what I will call Fart-X. Fart-X? Wasn't that one of the robot leads in Star Wars? No way! I'm not taking anything that might launch me out of bed in the middle of the night and bounce me around the walls on one of my trips to the bathroom. How could anyone, any sane person, stare at a bottle called Fart-X and drink it? But I did, and it did, and the surgery went well. Well, that's what I was told because one of the great advantages of surgery is that for the first time in years, I had uninterrupted sleep.

I was given my medications and instructions about when and how to take them that my wife wrote down because even on a good day, I wouldn't remember. But I did notice that the nurse was wearing a radiation detector. Are you joking? Who are those other people wearing white plastic suits with hoods covering their heads, peering through clear visors and breathing through oxygen masks? Why are you releasing me back into the world? No, you'll be okay, I was told. Just don't hold a newborn too close. How about airport security? Don't travel right away. What if I get stopped in the New York subways and the police scan me? They'll arrest you and you'll explain … Big deal. Have them contact our call center in the Philippines during business hours. There is a toll-free number to our hotline next to the organ donor release that we hope you will sign.

Next, the nurse gave me a stool softener. Little did I know how much I would need it, nor how ineffective it would be. And true to its label, within three days I was constipated. I didn't want to go to the emergency room, but my wife insisted. So, after holding out until midnight and testing the limits, once again, of our marriage, I went. Luckily, it wasn't busy. I was ushered into a private room where a PA greeted me. A PA, for those of us who are uninformed, is a Physician's Assistant, or an "almost" doctor. Doctors don't treat their patients at the hospital anymore. The PA's do it. The "Hospitalists" do it. A what? Hospitalist? Isn't that the title of daytime drama for the chronically bored? Needless to say, no one does house calls anymore, if you are old enough to remember what those were. If you want your doctor to actually come to the hospital or, at least, promise to come, then you have to pay a premium for such service. Are you out of your fucking mind? I'm going to sign up for "concierge service" at $2000 a year to see my own doctor? I quit that primary care physician's group immediately. Did he care? No. He wasn't going to make any money on me anyway. So I fired him very loudly in the waiting room filled with two-dozen people. Did anyone beg me to come back? No.

I explained my problem to the PA: I haven't had or been able to have a bowel movement in three days. Not that I didn't try or want one, or wish to spend some quality time with my oncologist. The PA gave me a laxative that, after a half-hour, had no effect. When she came back into to my curtained little room and found me staring up at a TV that didn't have a very good selection of cable channels, or any channels for that matter, I was craning my neck upward to a corner of the ceiling that induced airsickness, and she could smell the results immediately. I was beginning to give off a very unpleasant odor. My apologies, once again, to my wife. The PA asked me to turn over and she stuck her finger you know where. Oh, my. I forgot what I was missing. My rectum was clear. This is **good** news? I haven't had a bowel movement in three days. Whatever I ate must be somewhere. She kindly informed me that my colon was impacted. I just had prostate surgery and was about to go nuclear. I was officially a dirty bomb. But the most fun was yet to come. She gave me a stronger laxative and said that if nothing happened in thirty minutes, she would have to do a "digital" disimpaction. Certainly, you're kidding. I took out my iPhone and waved it in front of her. "**Digital**, as in there's an app for that I can purchase from the iTunes store?" She smiled and raised a single finger … her middle finger. "Digital" disimpaction. She was going to stick her finger back up to what was now being confirmed in my mind as the medical comfort zone and, in the tradition of all great doctors and auto mechanics, release me manually. Release me. Manually. What am I now? Man up. Or in the language or Old Brooklyn where I grew up: Go Fuck Yourself!

"Is this your dream job?" I asked the PA, as my wife turned away in a ritual she had become used to since we were married.

"Well," the PA began and thought about it with a fine sense of her profession and mission in life: "Yes, it is my dream job. Not my dream procedure." She smiled. "Not yours, either. I promise." Toodle-loo. "I'll be back in a little while. Don't go too far."

This time I gulped down magnesium citrate and

now I was getting weak.

"Everything all right, hon?" asked a nurse asked from outside the closed curtain.

"I'm fine," I answered, as my wife opened the curtain for a peek.

"She's speaking to someone else down the hall."

"Oh." The phone rang at the nurse's station and I picked up my phone. I was so sleep deprived that, earlier in the day, I put the wash in the machine, added the detergent and forgot to run the cycle. But I didn't forget to take it out and put it into the dryer.

Finally, at about 3 AM, we both wanted to go home. We packed up, got into the car, and a sudden gurgling sensation began to take over my whole being, so we flew through red lights. Magnesium citrate can launch a space shuttle. Seconds after we pulled into the driveway, I unlocked the back door to the house so no one would notice us coming in and bounded carefully up the stairs. My body exploded just as I hit the toilet. And continued to do so for another three hours. Thank you, thank you … Thank you. At least magnesium citrate was lemon flavored. Now I have a fresh bottle sitting in our liquor cabinet next to the Margarita mixes for our next party. Cocktails anyone?

CHAPTER THREE

Every Day is a Gift

For a week or so, I felt no difference. I was fine. I even slept a whole night with a catheter attached. Wow! This made the procedure almost worthwhile. Of course, I would have to wear it in certain public places, but who would know? I was actually warming up to it, but eventually I would have to terminate our growing intimate relationship and take the catheter out. This was a bit of a negotiation, but I managed to cut it, deflate the balloon inside me and wiggle it out painlessly. Phew! No shooting stars, no volcanic eruptions or nuclear reactions. I had been told that the seeds would start to heat up within two to four weeks, so I waited with great expectations. But … How does one feel when the inside of your body is becoming radioactive? Do you expel burning beads of luminescent perspiration? Do you disgorge heat-seeking pellets? Do your eyes glow? The doctors told me what they knew from studies and the experience of other patients. Statistics. As we all know, however, unless, the doctors have gone through the same procedures, it's all third party information—and I was the third party. Nevertheless, I was treated with great care and sensitivity. I was also a wealth of personal validation and, having had next to no sleep, I managed to stumble into the doctor's office for my next visit.

"You look tired," my urologist said.

"Really? I had a full 45 minutes of sleep last night."

Think about it. You don't sleep. You struggle through a restless night of discomfort, crush your toes in the dark on your way to the bathroom and … You are rewarded by waking up early. Real early. I'm talking 3 or 4 AM. So what do you do? Stay in bed and stare up at the ceiling? Turn on the TV? No, not me. I got out of bed, went to my computer and wrote for a couple of hours. No, not this book. Although I had been keeping a journal, this one took 5 months before I could put a word on paper and then I put it aside for a few years to gain perspective on how cancer was affecting my future and, in many ways, forcing me to relive events of my past. Yet, prostate cancer is invisible. No one knows you have it unless you reveal it. You don't lose your hair, you don't announce your presence physically with masks and tubes, and you are not quarantined. But it is very definitely with you because prostate cancer affects you privately.

Many details of what you do every day, ones that barely register when you are healthy because there is no reason to think about them, come into focus and the word "cancer" becomes a very new, but real part of the present. Is a bold lettered word that you must add to your vocabulary. At first it is in the form of questions to yourself: Go to a movie? Can't sit that long. Take a walk on the beach, or even down the street? How long will I last? Read a book? Maybe you can't because you just don't have the strength. Take a car ride? Don't go too far from the bathroom. Travel? Is there a hospital near by? I still had much to learn about the experience and I kept returning to the past through the journal I kept at that time when my father was being treated for cancer.

I still had to teach, however; but no one had any idea I was being treated for cancer. I was also commissioned to write a play just before my diagnosis. The teaching had to continue and the play had to be finished. Little did the director and cast know that they would have to go through more than a dozen drafts because nothing was coming out right from pellets to prose. At least I had something to do during my waking hours, which was pretty much all night; and the time before the phone starts ringing is a very good time to be creative. So, as sleepless as I was, I channeled the energy that would be sapped from me all day long into my imagination and my imagination onto the page. I ignored the discomfort and accepted the frequent urgency to go to the bathroom. In spite of these trips every fifteen minutes, I worked on the play and another book I was editing. There was no time for me to feel sorry for myself. My father would never allow it for himself or me because the future was clear, as my father told me after he died the first time. Yes, **after** he died the first time on the operating table when his leg was being amputated for a blood clot, and years before prostate cancer finally took his last breath. His simple, but profound words are always with me: "Every day is a gift." And I never forgot them.

What had finally given him eternal peace had provided new energy and spirit to me. I would try to be as creative as I could: write, teach, and take a nap when I couldn't focus any longer or because I couldn't doze off for more than thirty minutes at a time. If I had nothing else to show for the aches, pains, anxiety and distress, I had transformed a blank page into a creative work of drama. I had changed an empty space into the three dimensions of theater. I had created something that lived and breathed where nothing existed before; and I did it in the spirit of my father who was always positive, never gave up, and maintained his smile and sense of humor until his last comforting look.

This is how I remember final moments by his side as my wife held his hand. Everyone else had stepped out of the hospital room or found a space nearby to get themselves comfortable for a few hours of sleep during a long night, but I wouldn't leave him, and neither would my wife. I was wearing a gold ring with a brilliant opal that my grandfather had given to him and he had given to me, and I took his other hand in mine. His grip tightened as he tilted his head slightly to acknowledge my presence, and I leaned closer. His eyes became lucid—serene—and seconds later, before everyone else had come too late to his bedside, he died in peace. Even though he lives within me now and inspires my life, his passing would take years to come.

CHAPTER FOUR

Cancer is Not a Communicable Disease

Cancer is not infectious. You can't catch it in public like a cold from someone next to you. It is also not communicable, as defined by most of us who find cancer extremely difficult to talk about. Medical professionals speak in clinical terms and statistics; family and friends speak in hushed, protective tones if they can find the words. When they are forthcoming, they are often afraid, choked up and, after a prolonged illness, sad or philosophical about it. Occasionally they are brutal, as if the person who has been overcome with cancer somehow did it on purpose—not just to him or herself—but to the spouse, family, and friends. Often, they are guilt ridden: What did I do to deserve this? I'm sorry for putting all of you through this. I should have … I never should have …Why me? Why me!

The pressures are too great, the responsibilities

enormous, and sometimes the response to cancer is thoughtless or offensive with a devastating impact. One woman who claimed to be a "good" friend of my father's, as if I didn't know my father's good friends, stopped me in the hospital hall on my way to see him as she was leaving from a brief visit. With great authority and a sense of self-importance that she was offering comfort and support, she told me: "These things take a while."

These things take a while. Even now, I wonder how someone can be so callous. But she did not hesitate to lecture me on how long death takes.

I stared at her, but she wasn't satisfied with her offense and could not control the urge to assert her proprietary relationship with my father and unfiltered superficiality to make the inevitable easier on me. Reassuringly, she added: "He left you a nice legacy."

I drilled her with my eyes: Fuck you!

She walked away without another word.

She was right, however, on both counts. His death was long and painful, and in her pettiness and self-centered opinion of herself, she had no idea how deeply his legacy affected so many people.

• • •

As a teenager, my father was not just a father to me. He was a father to many of my friends on our block in our tightly knit Brooklyn neighborhood where we left our doors unlocked and shared our front porches with a cup of coffee, a Coke, or a beer, sometimes talking to neighbors across the street from one porch to another. My friends would come over to our house day or night whenever they wished, walk up the front porch and into the living room. Then they settled down, or went directly into the kitchen, our community gathering place for conversation. If I were home at the time, they would ask if they could speak to my father and it would be simple: "Dad, Billy's here and would like to talk to you." I would go get my father and leave them to their private conversation.

This is how people remember Benson Meth. He would welcome my friends to join him on the front steps of the house in warm weather. He would hold court in the screened-in back porch near our makeshift basketball backboard where my friends came to shoot for as long as they wanted because we had the only backboard on the street. He listened attentively and patiently to their concerns and problems about issues they were uncomfortable talking about with their own parents. Their personal concerns may not have been solved, but my friends were satisfied that they could speak to my father, a person who would give them the time and maybe some advice, but not judge them.

It was during these early teenage years that my father began to develop serious health problems, and they didn't come gradually, but with a thud. I was with him as often as possible during his many, many days in the hospital because of a blood clot in his calf and repeated attempts by the doctors to save a leg that was becoming numb from the knee down. He even joked about it as if it weren't part of his body, until it wasn't. As much as I loved him, I could not get him to realize that he was not protecting me by pretending that his health wasn't in jeopardy. He imagined that by showing me he was not worried, there was nothing to worry about.

One afternoon, when I came into the hospital after school, he was sitting up in the hospital bed reading a newspaper after a failed attempt at replacing part of a vein with a pig's vein. His leg was raised up on a pillow and he invited me to touch it, as if it were not part of his body, but an amusement. I shuddered. It was turning blue and just out of the freezer, ice cold. My father, however, was matter of fact about it: Remove it. Big deal. The touch, the iciness, even the vision is easy to recall to this day; but as a young teenager, what could I do? I stayed by his side during these very troubling times, but it was something he refused to acknowledge because he thought it was all going away.

Then the day came. I had just returned home from school and walked into the living room where my mother was on the phone with the hospital. The way she looked at me made me confused. It could not be good news.

"Your father died."

Question marks. Exclamation marks. Tears.

His heart had stopped. My heart stopped. He died on the operating table and I felt a terrible, deep sadness and … No, this could not be! I didn't know what to do or who to turn to. After all, my father was the man whom all my friends came to when they couldn't speak to their own parents. Now he was dead. Who would I speak to now? How would we survive? I couldn't imagine it. He was gone.

I couldn't sit. I couldn't stand still. I couldn't breathe. Then there was another call and my mother's voice lowered.

"What?"

I tried to get some idea of what she was hearing, but my mother's face was changing and, once again, I was confused.

"It's the surgeon."

"What?"

"Your father's alive."

"Daddy's alive?"

"He opened your father's chest, massaged his heart and brought your father back to life!"

I didn't stop to imagine that this was a miracle. All I could think of was that my father was not leaving us.

It took my father a long time to talk about this experience, but there was something, I would later learn, that my father wanted to tell me.

From the day he left the hospital and returned home, he was more determined than ever to succeed. He had lost at least thirty pounds, his strength was sapped, the muscle sagged from his arms and legs, and he was barely able to move. He was fragile but his spirit was indomitable. It was difficult for him to walk from the upstairs bedroom, downstairs to the living room and kitchen, and back again when he had to go to the bathroom. But he did it many times each day. It was a routine that we had all taken for granted until we watched my father struggle with the easiest of chores.

Then I heard it: A crack. A single, dull pounding sound. As my father made his way awkwardly upstairs to the bathroom, I ran from the kitchen and found him on the floor. One of his wooden crutches had snapped and I couldn't get to him fast enough, as he lay sprawled on the second landing. I helped him off the floor, got a spare pair of crutches and, although he wasn't hurt, he was angry with himself for falling and being too weak to stand up on his own. But he was okay.

Later that night when we were all in bed, I heard the crutches snap again and ran down the stairs to the kitchen from the converted attic where I slept. My mother came out of the bedroom first to see what had happened.

"Dad!" I yelled.

"David, what?" my mother asked.

"I heard daddy's crutch break," I said and looked around for him.

"I'm all right, my son," he assured me as he came out of the bedroom.

It was a nightmare … One that I would have for many years.

• • •

He hadn't been back to work, but by his bedside was a huge, fun, hand-made get-well card with the signatures of all the people in his office wishing him a smooth and uninterrupted recovery. It was a card that I would look at and reread many times as I sat by the bedside or watched as he did what primitive exercises he thought would restore his health and strength in a slow but steady way. There was something else occurring, however, that he would recover from more quickly than I. He did not know it, but my mother was having an affair with his best friend while he was in intensive care. I was aware of something without knowing exactly what it was at the time, but kids can sense there is something wrong between parents or in a family relationship without being able to identify it.

I never left my mother alone with my father's friend at the kitchen table, even during school nights. They never asked me to leave the room so they could be alone because they didn't want to reveal my suspicions about them or their guilt about what they thought I knew they were doing. It lay buried in our past for many decades until she died and I never said a word; but hidden behind a hesitant expression of dutiful affection by my mother, a phony smile, or a superficial greeting, the knowledge we both shared was never uttered in words, but the emotions could hardly be concealed:

"How are you, honey?" my mother would say when I came back from school.

"Fine, mom."

"Everything okay?" she added without particular reason.

"Sure. Why?"

"Just asking."

Just festering.

CHAPTER FIVE

The Time I Died

My father was never a person to make an issue of his situation no matter how difficult it was. During his many hospitalizations, the loss of his leg and his death on the operating table, he considered himself lucky and felt grateful to be alive. When he received the massive, very heavy, awkward wooden prosthetic tree stump that was cut to look like a leg, it gave him a great deal of pain for many months until he developed enough callous so it wouldn't hurt him as it rubbed against the bone. He walked to the subway station every day with visible effort as he had to lift his whole leg to take each step, but he continued to go dancing and look for a new partner. Of course, he had no choice because my mother wanted to begin a new life and divorced him about a year after the surgeon had brought him back to her life. Without another word, ever again, it became clear as the years went by what she had been hoping for.

I don't know what was going through my father's

mind, but he never faltered or blamed himself for the divorce. The divorce was over and done, and the limp was now part of his life. He was never bitter as he wrapped the stump below his knee in layers of thick cotton socks as a daily reminder that he had other goals and he would not be stopped. He was never well balanced; yet, he was pleased by the fact that he was mobile and could drive to go out on dates in his 40's. His lessons were my lessons, and he taught me never to consider myself a victim of circumstance or illness because there were no negatives in his life. He would make the best of any situation. So would I.

• • •

One day, I met him at the BMT subway station on East 14th Street and Ave. H, as I liked to do when he returned from work. We would get a Coke or a cup of coffee at Bernie's Candy Store or just walk home together. Sometimes during the late days of spring and summer, he would stop at the dead end where we were playing stickball and he would watch the game with other fathers and people returning from work. When the game was over, he and I would walk home together and catch up on each other's day. My father and I just liked being together, a bond that needed no reason or explanation. As we were walking down East 14th street, a local neighbor passed by and my father asked how he was.

"I'm old," he said, looking at my father for sympathy. "We can't expect much from life at our age," he added. "After all, I'm 45."

My father lifted up his pants' leg and knocked on the wood.

"I've never felt better," my father said. "Stop complaining and go home."

The man walked on, embarrassed and hurt that my father would speak to him so unsympathetically. Couldn't my father understand? My father paused for a moment, took out a cigarette and lit it. 'David, my son, I want to tell you about the time I died."

He said he was heavily sedated, but described the experience as if he were a bystander looking on, watching himself from above. He told me how he had been called before an omnipotent being who was sitting in a very high chair like the one Lincoln's statue sat on in Washington, D.C. My father's time had come, he was told and, quite simply, he said no. This higher being asked him how he could refuse. It wasn't his decision to make. Why should he be given another chance? My father didn't hesitate for moment and explained that he was not negotiable: He wanted to see his three sons get a good education, grow up, get married, raise their own families, and become successful. My father was not about to be granted his wish, nor be allowed to negotiate. My father's fate was sealed, and this superior being was very clear: He had heard my father's response many times before from many other people. What makes you special my father was asked. It didn't matter. My father refused to die. He didn't use the word God to describe this encounter, but he said, "David, my son, every day is a gift."

<u>CHAPTER SIX</u>

Ideal Circumstances

One of my father's early gifts was an idea that he developed in the early 1960s, and it was brilliant considering there were no personal computers or Internet access at that time. He still had to work full-time and we were partners on his way to one of his many dreams: a new business called Source of Supply. Armed and feeling quite important with the acronym SOS, I went down to Brooklyn Borough Hall every Monday through Friday and copied the names and contact information for all the new businesses registered and meticulously written in beautiful penmanship in the public ledgers the previous day. Later that night, my father typed them on a mimeograph stencil and ran them manually through this low cost printing process to mail copies to his growing number of paid subscribers. The guarantee: They would be the first to offer their services or products to these new businesses. Perfect. Until I got too busy with school and my own part time work and had to stop.

My father continued to speak to people, look for new employment possibilities, and send out his resume. Then it happened: He was offered a new job with a promotion and a better salary at the Pitney Bowes Corporation in Stamford, CT at a time when you could see the Long Island Sound from I-95. He was going to leave Liggett & Myers Tobacco Company where he worked and smoked two packs of cigarettes a day because in the Sixties smoking was what everyone did and no one thought twice about it except when they needed a light. Cancer? That happened to other people and even then it was barely a topic of conversation. In spite of the immense and serious health problems he had just been through, going for an annual check up never entered his mind because he was now free; and freedom meant moving to Connecticut

Freedom did not quite have the same meaning for me, however, as I was about to embark on the second most significant change in my life. The first was in living without my family as I stood frozen at the steps of our front door and watched my mother leave with my brothers and walk down the street to their new home, a large studio apartment with barely enough room for them, no less me. It may as well have been California. They were gone. My family was over. The next change was in adjusting to living with a new family: My father was getting remarried to a very attractive woman with a full head of red hair and blue eyes who brought immediate attention to herself, especially when she approached my bedroom in Brooklyn, looked at my wall of books and said, "This won't do. You can't bring those to my house." Her house.

This declaration was coming from a person whom I never had a problem with while she and my father were dating for a year or so. I actually liked her until this first stark moment that froze the reality of what was to come, although I had no idea how thin this icy surface would become and how we would sink below it ... except for my father.

Her eyes, which at times could exude warmth and welcome, penetrated anyone who put her on defensive alert: No compromise, no backing down. Test me.

Unfortunately for this new social arrangement, I, too, did not back down. Yet, survival dictated that the transition had to be one of compromise from everyone involved. To prepare me, my father invited her son to our house. When he called out to introduce him, because … Where exactly was he? I was greeted by a resounding "Huh …?" from deep inside our refrigerator, an expression that evoked an overstuffed mouthful of Twinkies and tended to ring in your ears long after the voice was gone. Then he materialized: a 16-year old, pear shaped creation who had very short hair and Mister Potato Head ears whom she all but petted and purred over. In spite of how he was the antithesis of everything she wanted everyone to believe him to be, I was required to accept him as my brother. Oh, really? My father, however, extended his love and welcomed him as one of our family as he did with all my friends. The word "brother" never left his lips.

An unmovable, unbreakable wall of tension began to form immediately. In asserting her authority, my father's new bride would make every attempt to break the bond between my father and me because they were now husband and wife and her son and I were "brothers," equals, and we had to adjust. Well, I was older, so I had to adjust: my work schedule, where I placed my food in the refrigerator for later at work so he wouldn't bite into the center and leave it; my weekend schedule: I escaped to the City. Thus, our idyllic beginning together went on for two years of unmitigated agony during which my father would sit down with me in private to defend his marriage and explain that he loved his second wife and that her son also needed a father. But why was there never mention of his father? The question always lingered, but it was never broached: How did he come to be?

My lack of acknowledgement of her son; my disavowal of him with a barely raised eyebrow was something she could not tolerate, and her volatile behavior began to appear in spurts. At first, I attributed it to four people in quarters that were too close trying to get used to each other for the first time. But there was too much anger and emotion because it was difficult to reason without an explosion of indignity, outrage, and hurt feelings that she constantly accused my father and me of causing. Sometimes my father would take me aside and ask me to have patience with her son who was the clinical definition of "gross" and created new meaning for the word "obnoxious." Yet, my father was always available as his father.

It was difficult and at times mockingly funny, especially when her loving human pet stranded her in the airport lounge one day to watch the end of a football game on a small pay per view TV. When I asked my father where they were, he barely had enough time to shake his head, "No" and say, "Don't say a word," before the front door opened. "Was there a lot of traffic?" I asked naively and became the recipient of one of her withering stares and challenges to a blistering battle that she was ready to inflict on me instead of her son.

Life for the four of us continued to be the subject of many discussions between my father and me and I understood his willingness to keep trying and remain committed to the woman he married and said he loved. But he never had an answer when I asked him why he would stay with a woman who was becoming more and more abusive. It finally came to a point when he had to force himself to give me an ultimatum that he knew I would understand, and he did it very gently with great love and affection: I would have to change and adapt or leave. But it was a forgone conclusion that we both didn't need to acknowledge because I was planning to move back to the city to continue my college education and the next stage of my life. It was painful for him to say because such a decision was not imposed on her son who was still in high school and who had no other father figure in his life. Intolerable as each day was, I was not ready to leave, and although I didn't tell him, I was not ready to abandon my father in spite of his unwavering positive attitude.

CHAPTER SEVEN

Survival

I drove back to Brooklyn every weekend where I spent time and let out my frustrations and anger with my friends Danny, Roy, and Zev. During my father's illnesses, from the time his leg was amputated, his divorce from my mother, and the second marriage, I had lost control of my life. But my very close friends, all who had a special relationship with my father, stood by me. Without Danny and Roy, I would not have survived my mother's infidelity, the profound loneliness of separation from my brothers with the break up of my family, and my father's second marriage.

After school and late into the night, I would slam the cue ball into a rack of balls battered by the problems of so many other teenagers in Arty's poolroom. I vented my frustrations to my friend Roy who shared my father's love, too. He like, Danny, was at my house as if it were his own. His father had died just before he entered high school and we all found ourselves trying to understand each other's lives at a time when not all parents were available or welcoming. Sometimes I sat yelling for hours in one of Danny's rented rooms, and later in my used car that I had saved up for working part time and bought for $500.00. Danny listened patiently and waited until I calmed down before we went into Bernie's Candy Store for coffee. Danny could understand. His stepfather, a truck driver, had thrown him out of the house when he told him he was planning to go to college. Danny had his own special relationship with my father, who loved him, too, and he moved into our house after moving from one local boarding house to another.

And then I met Zev. I was 17 and he was 16 and had just emigrated from Israel. He looked older than he was, and I, with a neatly cropped full beard disguised my young age easily. So it was not difficult to get into all the discos and nightclubs that would not admit anyone under 21. I was never even asked for I.D. Neither was Zev, because wherever he went, he brought his friends and beautiful young women. We all made our grand entrance walking into the Ginza, one of the most popular clubs of the time. Entering with Zev, however, was an experience in a category of its own and everyone wanted to share it. As we came down the open stairs from the street level entrance to the dance floor below, there was a hush. People whispered Zev's name. Women dropped their dates and various articles of clothing, and lined up to grab him onto the dance floor. The men wanted to be with Zev and wear one of his ornately styled, high gold rings that he made as a young jewelry designer. To show off your custom designed ring was to announce to everyone that you were a friend of Zev's, that you were special because he was special and loved by everyone. He was uniquely handsome and charismatic, and to be in his wake, to catch the overflow of the beautiful women who followed him and vied for his attention was a thrill and, of course, a goal. Yet, he was a kind, unpretentious person with a generous smile who welcomed everyone and was welcomed as a member of my extended family with Danny and Roy. .

From our later years in high school and into college, our small group went from long Sunday brunches at my house to a nearby luncheonette, a local dive with greasy bacon and eggs, English muffins dripping with butter, and endless cups of coffee to wash down the Vietnam

War, the Civil Rights Movement, and Rock n' Roll in a three-inch thick Sunday New York Times. We sat together and tried to work out our personal troubles, as well as the problems of the world in the Sixties, and the events became narrative threads for very dramatic and dark, but sarcastically funny stories. Being completely open to each other and sharing our lives kept us as balanced as teenagers could be. None of us knew where our future would take us at that point in time, but we all had the sense that together we were forever.

CHAPTER EIGHT

Evicted

After more years in Stamford at a job that he had mastered within months and that he could do without effort, my father could not go any higher within the corporation. He went into work and was at his desk by 8AM, delegated his staff's responsibilities by 9AM, and had little to do for the rest of the day. Once again, he wanted to establish his own business; but this time he created an independent consulting firm for international transportation, the profession he had gained a great deal of expertise in. Together, the second wife who hated every minute of helping him and my wife and I would go with him to the conferences he had set up at hotels in and around the local area. At these two-day seminars, people in the profession would attend classes and lectures and upon completion would receive a certificate certifying that they had studied with Benson Meth at the Connecticut Institute for International Traffic. It was shortly after his dream was being fulfilled that he was diagnosed with cancer. His condition deteriorated rapidly over the next two years. So did our superficial second family that had no roots except in dreams for a new beginning. The frail relationships we had frayed quickly and broke down, communication was inadequate and painful, and this seventeen-year trial was over.

But the second wife was never at a loss for words that flowed freely and viciously. She was a woman who despised men and especially her father. Her first marriage, if she had been married before, gave birth to her only son, and was a subject my father would not talk about it, except to reiterate that she had been terribly abused. Both her mother and her sister had profound mental illness. Her mother lived out her life in an asylum and her sister committed suicide. As a result, this woman whom my father said he truly loved used every opportunity to vilify him in the most ugly and provocative terms. During those rare moments when she was not totally absent of heart and self-destructive and we could enjoy the evanescent present, she could sometimes be pleasant with a delightful sense of humor and a hearty laugh. We actually had some fun times together with fall-on-the-floor belly laughs. But she turned on the slightest perceived indignity or imagined provocation and berated my father, my brothers and me, with complete disregard for anyone else present. Yet, when I challenged her about her behavior, she looked at me genuinely shocked as if I were talking about someone else.

"I would never do such a thing," she said when I repeated some of her vile words. "I would never say that."

When I confronted her with exactly what she said, she denied it and was deeply hurt because it could not be her. Yet, people began to stay away from my father and her when they were together. Rarely could they find dinner companions and were left to themselves except when my wife and I came up.

My father's cancer diagnosis put her over the edge and his two-year deterioration empowered her with a sense of cruelty that was unimaginable. On the one hand, she evoked sympathy that my father, no matter how much suffering he endured, always made an effort to give because he knew what she had endured early in her life. But it was never discussed and it was apparent deep down inside her that she was possessed by loneliness and insecurity. But how much abuse can be tolerated? As the intensity of her verbal and psychological assaults grew, I learned what it felt like to want to do violence to someone and I told her that if I had a baseball bat I would crush her face. I told her that in front of my father who was bedridden and in tears. Her response: Go ahead. See what happens. It was difficult to control myself, so I kept a journal. If I couldn't control the situation in my daily life, at least I could write it out of my entire being.

• • •

Emotions were volatile and unpredictable because the cures for cancer at that time were worse than the disease and no one knew how to talk about it. My father did not complain about his constant discomfort, but it took only one look at him, a short visit, to realize that he would not be cured. Everything he ate, he threw up; his body was always in pain, and his medications interfered with each other.

But the second wife resented my father for putting her through this terrible ordeal. She also didn't want to be left on her own. How do you deal with a person who evokes sympathy but becomes heartless at the same time? My wife tried her best to keep her from disintegrating further and spent time alone with her in her antiques shop. But she was out of control and unbearable, so my wife had to limit her time with her because she constantly berated my father. Eventually she had to stay away.

My father's only solace was to move to a full care nursing facility, but not out of his own volition. If he was going to die, it wasn't going to be in the comfort and familiarity of his own home. At his new residence, at least the abuse would stop. It was both a relief and a new fact of life that was difficult to adjust to: the second wife had forced him to leave, but she was far from done. As unpredictable as this woman could be, she would assert a proprietary right in the future that was, by any stretch of the imagination, inconceivable. It would also be irrevocable.

• • •

It is difficult, even today, in looking back over my journal to describe how I felt on my first visit to what was then called a "nursing home." My father was set up in a wheel chair and accepted this turn of events, as if he had moved to a new office. With pencil in hand and a yellow pad, it was as if he were going to continue doing business from his bedside. But all of the people he had trained and to whom he now offered to sell his business stole his clients when they were certain he wasn't coming back to work.

I looked forward to my visits with him and took him for a stroll in the wheelchair. He introduced me to some of his new friends and all was peaceful and quiet and went well until I had to say good-bye that first visit. I kissed him and told him that I would be back in a day or so; but when I got outside the front door of the facility, I couldn't move and turned back to stare at the entrance. How could I leave my father this way? How could this woman whom he was married to for 17 excruciating years evict him from his own house?

This is the way cancer infects the survivors around the cancer patient. The inability to deal with the fading loss of life, the profound memories of the past, and the denial of companionship, provoke feelings that are unrestrained. Communication is stilted, if it exists at all, and the expression of emotion takes over the expression of self.

A Bond

There is more information than ever about techniques and treatments for cancer that did not exist in the past and continue to expand and evolve. I have benefitted directly from these medical advancements, but the person who is diagnosed with cancer is still alone and it is still cancer. Concerned about what will happen if the condition deteriorates, the patient and loved ones find it difficult not to imagine the worst. The emotional investment and reaction to the word "cancer" and the look of dread that overcomes the people who say it or hear it is devastating. So I had to ask my urologist in considering whether I should proceed: With the news that the PSA test and numbers may be useless, and the side effects are debilitating and harmful, "What would you do if you had prostate cancer?" He was quiet for a moment. "I don't know," he answered honestly. Even he needed someone else to go to. That is why, perhaps, a friend called me after I had finished my treatment and asked if his friend could speak to me. He had the same diagnosis, and over coffee he confessed immediately: "I'm scared to death." I listened while he told me his concerns and asked me some questions about my experience. In some small way he felt comforted and less alone. Everybody needs support. Yet, most people are burdened by silence and feelings they are unable to express. The journal I kept during my father's illness and during my own, created a balance and left the experience, as I look back at it now, fresh in my mind.

However, for more than a decade after my father died I couldn't unclench my fist and I often had a recurring dream: My father was living in some dark, dismal apartment alone, unable to take care of himself, but he didn't want to burden me with care or concern and would not tell me where he was. The dream continued on an off, yet I did not have his phone number or any way to contact him. When I did have his phone number as part of the dream and called him, he told me not to worry, and that he was okay, but his voice was distant and he was alone. "David, my son," he said, "I love you" and told me he was going to hang up.

I couldn't get back to sleep, but the dial tone rang in my ears for years. One night, years later, however, my father came to me in a different dream and gently nudged my shoulder as he did often in the mornings to wake me up, sometimes with a cup of freshly brewed coffee to get me ready for school. This time he was with my grandfather and they assured me that everything was fine. It was good to see my grandfather. It was reassuring to be together with both of them sharing a bond that transcended time, distance and death.

• • •

In my early twenties after I left Connecticut, I was living in New York City, working and attending college. I was out frequently on the weekends toward the end of the 60's with Zev. This was the era of bellbottoms and polyester shirts, wide lapels and long hair, and it was my personal refuge.

As I often did on weekends, I went to pick up Zev some time after 9:00 PM so we could go into the City. I pulled up to his house in an old used Chevy I had bought for $500 and left in the middle of Ocean Parkway when it finally died because I wanted to know what it was that always caused the unbelievable traffic jams that infuriated everyone caught in them. I removed the license plates and walked to the nearest public bus stop, smirking all the way. But this evening I walked into Zev's house and the living room was bustling like a Middle Eastern bazaar with siblings, parents, uncles and aunts talking and drinking Turkish coffee. I was greeted with hugs and kisses and the conversation always started the same way.

"David. How are you?"

"Great Mr. G. Hi, Mrs. G. Is Zev home?"

"Anybody see Zev?" his father asked.

"You see Zev?" his mother looked around the living room and asked.

"Zev?" filtered out from somewhere.

"Your brother," his mother said.

"No, I didn't see Zev." The response seemed to float in the air.

"You know where Zev is?" One of his brothers asked.

"Zev's home?" came from his sister.

"I don't know," someone said from behind a corner. "You know where Zev is?"

"David, you want some coffee?" his father asked.

"Sure, Mr. G."

He carved out of a block of something black and put

it into a cup, boiling hot, and my lips started to burn even before they got to the rim.

"Whew!" I took a sip. "Good coffee, Mr. G. A little strong. Okay, I'm going to see if Zev is around the neighborhood."

"Try the Kosher pizza place," his mother said.

"Yeah, he might be there," someone else added.

"Didn't he eat already?" another person echoed.

"Does Zev eat?" came another retort.

"When he's home," somebody yelled.

"When's that?" a voice responded.

I was now on full alert. The coffee was working. Thirty-minutes later, I returned.

"Zev, back, Mrs. G?"

"Where did he go?" his mother asked.

"He left?" his father asked.

Round two.

"Anybody see Zev?" his brother said.

"I don't know. You see Zev?" one more voice bellowed.

"Who?"

"What?"

"Your brother."

"Zev?"

"No. You know somebody else called your brother Zev?"

"Another cup of coffee, David?" Molten lava was bubbling over and Zev's father poured me another cup.

"Sure, Mr. G." I took a sip. "Ohhhh … kaaayyyy! Gotta go!" I said for no apparent reason other than my body was now in motion. "Maybe he's somewhere," I added, not knowing where somewhere was. 'I'll be back."

"Let us know if you find him," his mother said.

"Yup!" I raised my voice to hear myself think.

"When's the last time you saw him?" his father asked.

"Uh, I don't remember. Gotta go." My legs were moving toward the door.

Thirty-minutes later, I was back. Round three. The coffee was on the table and I was drawn to it like a heroin addict.

"Ohhhh, yeahhhh!" I said and started running in place almost immediately as I finished the cup.

"How about another dose?"

"Oh, I don't know Mr. G. I'm feeling a little jumpy," I said doing squats and push-ups and running in place. "Zev come back yet?"

"Zev?" said a familiar voice.

"Zev?" I said.

"Come back from where? Where was I?" said a voice in its underwear in front of the staircase that led upstairs.

"Zev's here," said another voice, either in my head or from one of the family. I couldn't distinguish.

"Hey, David, Zev's here," his sister informed me.

"Dave, Zev's here," another voice said.

"Zev, David's here." Who said that?

"Zev's here?" his father added. "You want some coffee, Zev?"

"You're here?" his mother said.

"I was upstairs sleeping. Where else would I be?"

I was sparring with Mohammed Ali, only no one else could see him. "Okay, you ready to go out?"

"Yeah. Give me a couple of minutes to shave and get dressed. Why don't you have a cup of coffee?"

"I don't think so. Okay. No. All right. Nah. Why not? God help me. You drive."

"I don't have a license," Zev said.

"No problem. Get on my back. I'll run."

• • •

That night, where the beat and rhythm of rock music engulfed the large square bar of Nepenthe and made the French bartender scream and squeak for supplies while the music exploded on the dance floor, I had an unsettling feeling around 1:00 AM. I was in the middle of a delightful, mindless conversation with a lovely young woman in a micro-mini dress that she couldn't sit in and delighted in dancing in as she undulated with the rhythm as we spoke, I excused myself and went over to the pay phone. I called my father who was in Florida with my grandfather in the hospital. As soon as he picked up the phone and said, "David, my son?" I knew.

"I had a strange feeling about grandpa," I said.

"He just died," my father answered and gave me a few brief details. "I'll call you tomorrow morning, my son. Good night."

I loved it when he called me, "David, my son."

When I woke up from that dream in which my grandfather, my father, and I were together, I felt a sense of relief and my fingers began to straighten. It took me a very long time before I could write about some of the other events in my father's life and mine. Reliving these memories and writing about them has allowed me to release myself from the hold of the past, but why does this healing take so long? Why didn't someone tell me how to deal with these events before? Because engaging in a conversation about cancer brings out emotions that are difficult to deal with and often painful. But talking is not enough. Sometimes you have to put your words on paper, even if they are never seen by anyone else, especially, perhaps, if they are never seen by anyone else. This makes the experience concrete and puts the writer in control.

CHAPTER TEN

The Everlasting Embrace

Cancer is so much more than a disease. It is a psychic connection to the ones you love. On June 4, 2001, I woke up in the middle of the night and my clock was staring at me sometime after midnight. I had just had a dream in which I was having dinner with Zev. Although I was living in New York and later in Connecticut after my father had remarried, my friends Zev, Danny, and Roy sustained me in spite of their own difficulties and without whom I could never have survived those early years.

Zev moved to Florida with his family some years later after he returned from Vietnam, met the woman he loved and got married; but we had stayed in touch, separated by war, careers, and the independent directions our lives eventually took. Despite the distance between us, our bond strengthened and our friendship continued to grow. After our dinner in the dream, we rose from the table to shake hands, and he embraced me in a deep, warm hug. But when I tried to step back to say good-bye, he was crying and wouldn't let go.

It had been almost a year since his annual trip north to visit us with his wife and three sons. He had been diagnosed with lung cancer and he wasn't traveling anymore since his first seven-hour dose of chemotherapy that caused a massive stroke, paralyzed one side of his body and blinded him. His life as he knew it had been wrenched from his grasp at the relatively young age of 53. For a man who had never smoked and worked very hard to provide for his family with a successful business that he had built over the years, the complete loss of control over everything in his life was devastating. He went from being an independent, energetic husband, father and businessman, to a person who could not see or use his hands and talents as a hair stylist and the owner of his own salon, to a victim of prior years and experiences that could not be understood, much less be justified. Now, he said, he couldn't figure out how to figure it out. Was it his exposure to Agent Orange during the Vietnam War? Was it because of the chemicals he had inhaled at work every day? Or was it because he had been treated with massive doses of chemo and released from the hospital too soon because the hospital needed the bed for the next patient? All they had to do was allow him to stay a few extra nights to be monitored, but they wouldn't. Or was it because his doctor and hospital were negligent? His wife tried to get answers. The doctor did not return her phone calls. The hospital remained unaccountable. Though his body was withering, Zev struggled to maintain his dignity and did not realize the strength of spirit he was passing on to wife and three sons and to me.

I was in contact with Zev every week. But the morning after my dream, I called him, and when no one picked up the phone, once again, I knew. The following evening, Zev's son returned my call. Lung cancer had taken a warm, wonderful and very special man—a very dear friend, someone whom everyone loved and wanted to be with, and it hurt profoundly. My wife and I took a flight out the next day to attend his funeral, and when I arrived at his home, Zev's spirit filled the house as we exchanged stories and personal experiences about him and with him. I sat down with his wife, who told me that the previous night Zev had called her and their sons into the bedroom and asked to be propped up in bed. Then, short of breath, he gently, yet firmly embraced each of them, one by one, to say his last good-bye. I was stunned. He had passed on at exactly the time we had our last embrace.

Sometimes it's as if Zev has never left. He appears in one of my dreams, ready to go dancing, or talk over coffee. I ask him where he's been, but he doesn't give me a clear answer. Then he's gone. Until the next dream.

Closure is difficult and sometimes we need help. Religion provides faith and rituals, and we find comfort in gathering together to grieve. But it is up to each individual to discover and renew that very special relationship with the spirit of the person who has "passed on" because the spirit never dies. For this is a delicate journey separating the past from the present and joining love and grief. We do not know when the journey will begin or how long it will last. We only know that, at some time, we may be among those on the pilgrimage.

CHAPTER ELEVEN

The Thrill of Survival

Cancer makes you think. It forces you to assess your life, past, present and future: What did I do wrong? What should I have done differently? What should I do now? And often, as if you have been singled out among all others, you ask yourself: What did I do to deserve this? Then you come to a bleak conclusion: Maybe it's too late. Everything is beyond your control. How do you deal with complex treatments and circumstances outlined by graphics and statistics in pamphlets, brochures, printouts and appointments with doctors and hospitals? The mounds of information are overwhelming and the details are incomprehensible. No matter how much information you have, no matter what anyone else says, your life is up to you. You have to take control of your emotions, manage your time and, yes, take another look at the person you thought you were. The texture of each day that was supposed to be your future becomes blurred because you are very sick; but you must stay positive, be productive and create each day anew. Then you ask yourself: How?

You can sit alone in front of the TV, or lie in bed at night and let the end of your life as you envision it close in on you—or you can free your thoughts and emotions from the darkest constraints of your illness and visualize the next day. Putting your thoughts, goals and dreams somewhere so you can see them doesn't just help you form a new tomorrow, it puts perspective on the past and clarifies events and relationships that you hold dear.

I have used writing to allay the worst that happened or that I could imagine in words so that I could understand and manage each day anew. Often, I tucked my words away in a notebook to revisit another time. I have changed my words, erased them, and deleted them. I have rewritten them and altered the shape and course of my life, because once your thoughts and emotions are released from your heart, you become free. The spirits of my father and Zev helped me to understand their deaths. Writing helped me to cleanse myself and appreciate life for the second time.

• • •

My prostate surgery had come two years after I was walking along the street with my wife in Soho, enjoying the beautiful weather and the excitement of people from all around the world delighting in New York life. I passed a homeless veteran sitting between two storefronts accepting donations, but didn't pay much attention to him. He was part of the New York scenery. I also wasn't watching where I was walking and slipped off a smooth, hard cobblestone curb onto the black asphalt of unyielding street traffic. It was one of those falls in which you watch yourself from above and say to the person falling: Put out your arms. Break your fall. Unfortunately, I wasn't listening. It was the other person falling. To my wife's horror, but not to her surprise, I tend to do things the hard way: I landed on my hip with my left leg perpendicular to my body. When asked about my ordeal in muted sympathetic terms by others, I had to admit: It was a great day.

This was New York City: I wasn't hit by a bicycle or struck by a cab. I was not run over by a bus. I ended up flat on my back on Prince Street on Memorial Day weekend, 2010, and even though I could barely move for half an hour, I managed to inch my way backwards onto the sidewalk near the homeless Vet while my wife went to get the car. Everyone nearby, or who passed by on this marvelous spring day in this great city, offered to help, give me water, or make a call for me. But my leg was dangling from my hip and I had the distinct feeling that it was going to separate from the rest of my body and I would be delivered to the hospital in two parts. I wouldn't let anyone touch me. When my wife pulled up to the curb with the car, the homeless veteran who had been wounded, hurt, and had no place to call home, gently and slowly helped me get off the ground. I rested on one of the plastic cartons he had been sitting on as he shifted the other he was using to display his medals and Special Forces cap. My leg dangled limply from whatever it was attached to on what used to be my hip, as he gently supported me and helped me maneuver into the car. Very carefully and with great pain, I lowered myself into the seat. I was, however, alive. And now I was actually comfortable. To my unknown friend, this selfless veteran, thank you so very much.

But my wife was beside herself when I insisted that we finish the shopping we had planned at Zabar's on the Upper West Side and not waste this splendid day by going straight back to Connecticut to the emergency room. When we finally got to the 2nd hospital (the first one said they couldn't see me for 5 hours), I was taken care of immediately. The surgery went well, and I was confident that I would heal without further complications because I was basically in good physical health. That day in Soho was truly a gift.

CHAPTER TWELVE

Freeing the Heart

The success and treatment for cancer is not just about medical treatment. It is as much about personal interaction and introspection. Sometimes it's easier to talk to a stranger than to the doctor. It can be more comforting to speak privately or in small groups where you share your concerns from a personal point of view, not a clinical one; and you can be candid because the person you are speaking to doesn't have an opinion about your life. But opening up in front of other people can be awkward and you may not want to be so forthcoming. Working alone and writing, on paper or on your computer, provides an access point, even if you don't consider yourself a "writer." I have been looking over the journal I kept during and after my father's illness and, although more than thirty years have passed, every word carries the weight of the moment. The journal served me well then because it allowed me to document events that were extremely frustrating and which I had little control over. I was able to put on paper what my wife, my family, and I were going through when it was moving too fast to make sense. As I reread and relive each moment in my journal, I find some of the same emotions returning, and my heartbeat heightens. I have to turn the page. Some things can't be changed, so you have to move on, as difficult as it may be. But you can write the wrongs.

I have taught writing to all ages and levels of students for many years and learned how thought provoking and deeply touching journals, personal essays, stories and plays can be. Sometimes, however, the act of writing some of your deepest emotions forces you to revisit these moments as if you were entering a darkened room in space with only one door. And then it locks from the outside. In one writing workshop I conducted, the emotion described was fear: fear in three parts: First is the fear of addressing how the writer feels about being diagnosed with cancer and learning of the options for treatment. Of course, the diagnosis does not just mean you have cancer, but that you must now assess who you are to yourself, your family and friends, and what your future portends. Second is the fear of revealing such intense and personal sentiments in writing and how much of what you write says about yourself: your character, your successes and failures and, as you close your eyes, your dreams. Third is the fear of the inescapable: You must be true to what you believe and how you feel; you must acknowledge your thoughts and experiences, try to understand your emotions and those of the people close to you, and decide how to deal with this totally new perspective on life.

Allowing the power and beauty of writing to emerge and learning how beneficial the writing process is has to be experienced to feel free. But there was one additional fear: the fear that someone else might read what your have written. This is a legitimate concern that encourages the writer to put unqualified trust in family and friends. After discussing these very significant issues, the workshop participants began their journal entries with enthusiasm and spoke about them with honesty and some tears.

Children and teens, especially, become much less inhibited when they discover they are able to express themselves privately on paper, and a new maturity is revealed as they deal with very sensitive and complex topics. Writing provides a means to bring out feelings and concerns about friendship, loneliness or bullying, and a parent who has a serious illness. Children often want to read their thoughts and stories aloud or perform them. For me, reading over my eulogy to my father and reliving the conversations with him and other family members is a reflection of those times, just as important now. How does this process benefit the person who has just learned he has cancer or affect the people close to him? It doesn't cure illness, but it lessens the burden.

I learned this when I began a playwriting program at a local "alternative" high school as a result of an artistic fellowship I received. The students, who were cast out of their original high schools and sometimes by their families out of their homes, or whose parents were in jail or in rehab found dramatic writing as a way to temporarily loosen themselves from the complexities and complications of their lives. Their writing, though unsophisticated, explored paths they could not take and imagine conversations and confrontations they dared not have. Words and drama provided an escape from the abuse and violence they experienced daily through drugs, sex and alcohol at home and on the streets by creating a world they could control. On a couple of occasions, the security guard rushed into the room because one student had written a dialogue in which he was confronting the character who played his father and threatened to kill him because he had abandoned him and his younger brother. A pen became a knife and his words were weapons, as he asked his father why he had left them. All of his sadness, tensions, and aggressions were released in the classroom instead of at home or on the street.

CHAPTER THIRTEEN

Discussion and Preparation

Many parents believe that what their children don't know doesn't hurt. They want them to go on with their lives as if whatever is going on in **their** lives is not really happening. The children may understand that a parent is seeing the doctor, but too many parents believe that the nature and gravity of their illness can be disguised or hidden. Such a situation occurred when the mother of two of my private students was diagnosed with the early stages of breast cancer. She had two boys, one in 6th grade and the other in 8th grade, and she was deeply concerned. She had told my wife that breast cancer was prominent among the women in her family and she imagined the worst. My wife put her in touch with a friend who had just gone through a radical mastectomy and breast reconstruction and was recovering well. Speaking to her provided some insight and camaraderie and she didn't feel alone.

An opportunity came up, however, to discuss cancer with the oldest boy when my doctor called me during our lesson. Both boys had been given some basic information, and the 6th grader was taking it well; but the older brother, who was more knowledgeable, seemed to be upset according to his mother. I took the call, something I would normally not do during a lesson, and discussed a few issues with the doctor to pique the boy's curiosity. My wife, who overheard me speaking, understood what I was doing and asked me a couple of questions after the call to raise the boy's awareness that I was discussing something serious. Rather than move on to the lesson, I decided to open up a discussion about my cancer, so that he might think, "Oh, Mr. Meth has cancer and he's doing well."

I explained to him what prostate cancer was, how I made my decision based on my father's history, how I would be treated, and what I expected my recovery would be like. Since I continued to teach him and his brother during the surgery and radiation, and after the treatment, I could discuss my progress with him. The most important point that I stressed, however, was that not all cancer is life threatening and is often curable. But the family must show their love and support for the person who has the disease. He listened attentively and we also looked at some graphics on the computer.

During a workshop of breast cancer survivors, one participant took a deep breath and said how difficult it was for her young teen daughter to accept the fact that her mother had cancer. Perhaps it was not that she couldn't accept it, as much as it was that she didn't know how to accept it. When this participant described her daughter's first encounter, she relayed the incident as if it were happening before her eyes at the exact moment when she appeared with a scarf around her head. In spite of the fact that she had tried to prepare her daughter for the effects of her treatment and her loss of hair, her daughter would not look at her. It took some time, but her daughter learned to understand her own feelings about her mother and then her mother's feelings. It also made us think about where children derive their strength from and how their perceptions of what they see sometimes can't be explained—that these perceptions must be digested so that they can understand them on their own.

Discussion and preparation are invaluable for

children in our age of advanced technology because children can access a great deal of the available resources online and learn what a parent or sibling is going through. They can also learn how to participate in the care because they can ask questions and feel empowered with this knowledge. Of course, such information was unavailable thirty years ago when my father had cancer, and the attitudes were too protective because the parents were not as knowledgeable or prepared as they are today. Now the boys were concerned, but not frightened. They felt they could understand the situation and that they could participate in their mother's care in some way. Their situation was under control. Children and teenagers must be given a part in the care of the ill parent or sibling, even a friend, to help them overcome their illness and get better. If not, there is guilt later in life about what they could have done or what they didn't do.

I came to learn this when I was about 15 and my father was in and out of the hospital because of the blood clot and bedridden for his very long recovery. I wanted to help, but there wasn't much I could do except to speak to him on the phone or be by his side when I wasn't in school. I am truly grateful that I was close to him, as the bond we already had became even stronger. There were also many things I wasn't told, not necessarily about the illness, but as a result of it … things that I discovered on my own. If the parents don't explain the situation clearly, or if the children believe the parents are withholding something from them, the issue will surface again in the future. If it remains unresolved, its presence becomes a hidden source of anxiety and misunderstanding.

CHAPTER FOURTEEN

Completely Honest

When my father's leg was amputated, his recovery was nothing short of a miracle. He wasn't put on a program of physical therapy at that time; and if there were such a program, he certainly didn't know about it. But he began to exercise on his own with 5lb. hand weights. His struggle after his first confrontation with death was one that I felt compelled to share because I wanted him to understand that I was with him then and forever. So when he nudged me gently early one morning after he had recovered and was on his way to work, he told me that he and my mother were getting divorced. She and my two younger brothers were going to move down the street. I could go with them, if I wished, because I was old enough to make my own decision; but before he could finish the rest of his sentence, I said, "I'm staying with you, Dad." It wasn't really a surprise to my father, but what he didn't know was that some of what had I had seen or sensed while my father was in the hospital, was never resolved. And then the impact came forcefully in the most disturbing manner after my father was on his way to recovery because he was faced with the telling me the truth or protecting himself with a lie—and he would never lie to me.

One evening, I went down to the basement to work out with my weights and I heard some shuffling in an adjacent small storage room. I walked inside and my father was there with an earphone in one ear that was attached to an alligator clip on a wire running down the wall. He looked at me solemnly, not because I had caught him doing anything wrong, but because he had to explain what he was doing. With words that must have been very awkward for him to say, he told me that he was listening to my mother talking to another man and making plans with him while he was at work. I didn't know how to respond, but in reality I did know: I had picked up one of the phone extensions at the same time as my mother and heard the same conversation on another day. I had not, however, told my father. She was still my mother and we lived in the same house, and I had no idea how to deal with this situation. So he offered me the earphone and I listened. It was true. Now what do I do with this information? I was so profoundly ashamed by my mother's betrayal of my father, my brothers, and myself, I could not even tell this to Danny and Roy who would soon learn that my mother was getting married to my father's best friend. They never said a word, but I am sure they could feel my humiliation and stood by me.

I took this embarrassment and anger with me to school where I felt that everyone knew because my parents were the first in the neighborhood to get divorced. I also hid it inside me when I went to Arty's Poolroom with Roy and vented my outrage as I slammed the balls into the pockets and off the table. Sometimes, I stayed there until closing at 1:00 AM on a school night because I didn't want to go home. Often I would sit with Danny in Bernie's Candy Store on cold winter days just talking, or in the tiny room he rented in the attic of a private house where giant, man-eating sunflowers loomed above the commuters on their way to the subway just up the street from mine. Zev would also listen patiently on our way to the discos or after on our way to the Foursome Diner in Brooklyn at 4AM as the indignity intensified. About a year later, when I was informed of my mother's wedding, I didn't want to attend, but my father encouraged me to accept the inevitable and go. I hugged and kissed my mother and shook my father's friend's hand to congratulate them on their marriage, but all I wanted to do was to wash my hands and leave. Instead, I stayed and watched everyone else who knew my father play along with smiles and wish them well. My father never said a bad word about my mother or mentioned the friend again, and I never spoke of it to him or to them. Long after my father died, however, he once again demonstrated his generous very spirit. My mother's second husband said he was being punished for his betrayal of my father and that was why he suffered from kidney failure and had to be on dialysis for many years. He died on my father's birthday. My father had forgiven him. I never did.

CHAPTER FIFTEEN

75¢ An Hour

How could my father whose vulnerability had confronted him with death wake up every morning with such a positive attitude? Perhaps it is because he knew that every day was his "gift," his second chance, and that he had done his best to set a positive example for his sons. How could this attitude not be infectious? When I revealed to my doctors that my father had died from prostate cancer they were concerned, but my wife felt reassured that I would recover well because we had caught the disease with an early diagnosis.

I was jolted at that moment in the Red Cross office, because I felt my life had changed; but never, not even for a moment, did I feel threatened. It's not that I didn't understand it was cancer and that cancer makes its own rules. The doctors could find something else, somewhere else; or it could take a turn for the worse and spread to other parts of my body without notice. But I believed the will to live a productive life supersedes illness and, even if the disease takes over, the spirit of survival is passed on and makes the people who receive your spirit stronger.

My father never felt sorry for himself, and that sustained me. He scrutinized his attempts to achieve his goals and always moved forward. "Failure" was not in my father's vocabulary. It was a temporary stop on the way to another goal and final achievement. Although he didn't take care of his health, and seems to have had fortune at his back in this regard, I learned from his naiveté to take care of myself. But we can't prevent heredity from playing forward into the future or know about all the toxins we inhale and eat. My father understood the dangers of smoking from the time he had complications with his blood circulation, but he was unwilling to stop smoking because of over-confidence and denial. He also never imagined he would get cancer and taught me a lesson very early on for which I am forever grateful.

One weekend when I was in 4th grade, my parents had gone out and taken my younger brother. I was alone with the telephone on the wall in case of emergency and the TV for company. Then I discovered an open pack of cigarettes. Well, I couldn't resist. After all, my father smoked. So I took a cigarette out of the pack, made an attempt to tamp it down on my wrist just I had seen my father do over and over again, and put it between my lips to test it out. It felt good and I felt truly cool. Like my dad. Then I tried to light it. When I could get a spark and the match lit, I let the cigarette sit between my lips for a few moments with the match to the tip. If my father can do it, I can do it. Nothing to it ... until I heard the door unlock and open.

"We're back!" my mother said.

Quickly I tried to put the cigarette out, but who knew how? So I threw it into the trash basket. A few moments later, my father came into my room.

"David, my son," he said with a touch of amusement and looked into the basket. "Everything okay?"

"Yes, dad." I didn't know what to do with my hands, and my eyes kept wandering to the wastebasket.

"Anything you want to tell me?" he asked.

"Who, me?" I said, as he sat down on my bed.

"What's that in the basket?"

"What basket?"

"That basket."

"Oh, that basket?"

"Were you smoking?" he asked without trying to catch me in a lie. He moistened his fingertips, removed the cigarette and squeezed the barely lit tip between his fingers as thin wisps of smoke began to emerge. "You want to have a cigarette with your daddy?" he said and smiled.

Really?

He took out a pack and tamped it down on his wrist. Then he tapped his wrist again. Wow! A cigarette popped up.

Man! I want to learn how to do that!

He offered it to me and I took it. He lit his cigarette and inhaled deeply until it filled his lungs. I lit mine, took a puff, and knew I was becoming a man. I exhaled immediately.

That's all there is to it?

"No, my son. That is not how you do it. You have to take a deep breath until the cigarette fills your lungs, and then you exhale." He did it again. Just like the commercials.

I inhaled as much of the cigarette as I could until I felt it burning inside me and coughed it up for the next five minutes, as my eyes became teary and my nose ran. I had to put the cigarette down.

"Let me show you again, my son," my father said, punctuating his lesson with another long drag. Deep inhale. Slow, drawn out exhale.

"No, thanks, Dad. I don't think I want to smoke."

He rubbed my head and left the room. I stayed as far away from cigarettes as I could, except in his presence, because he never stopped smoking morning, noon, or night, breakfast, lunch, or dinner, and it gave me excruciating headaches.

• • •

My father didn't make a point of telling me not to do something when he thought I could learn a more important lesson by myself. He listened to what I told him I wanted to do, and I always told him. He allowed me to make my own decisions in order to grow with confidence. This is why so many of my friends came over to speak to him. This time it was about smoking. Another time it was about work. Occasionally about girlfriends. After my parents divorced, I told my father that I had found a part-time job after school. I liked the idea of working for my own money so I didn't have to ask him for any, because he had very little left after alimony and supporting my mother and brothers; and I wanted to buy my own brand new, particularly old, mostly ready to be abandoned used car. He thought this was excellent because he wanted to see me become independent, and he asked what kind of job it was. When I told him I was going to wash dishes at a local hamburger joint, he smiled.

Good. I have his full support.

How much? 75 cents an hour … and … free dinner. A coke, too.

"Let me know how it goes, my son." He took a drag on his cigarette with a pleasant smile.

I began at 4 PM that first Friday night and washed thick, heavy dishes that you could throw against a wall and wouldn't break. I stooped over a very low, deep sink scrubbing them until my hands were water logged and raw. All I had to do now was to straighten up to stand. At least I would eat for free. My break came during a lull and I sat down at the counter and perused the menu with great interest.

"I'll take a …" I said, as the owner walked behind the counter to the grill.

He glanced over his shoulder and looked placidly at

me. "You'll take a burger and a Coke," he said, and gave me a dry, rock-hard burger, cold fries and a Coke. At least the Coke wasn't warm. Thanks.

When I finished for the night, some time after 10PM, he told me to come in at 4PM the next day. Thanks. No thanks. He barely noticed the door closing on my way out. My father was sitting in the kitchen, smoking and having a cup of coffee that I could smell on my way in, a ritual we had established so we could catch up on the day's or night's events, or just because ...

"Well, my son?" He smiled.

"Don't think I'll be going back there."

"Oh?" His smile was warm with anticipation to let me know that he understood.

"He gave me a stale burger and cold fries. Plus, I broke my back. I just want to go to sleep."

"What did you learn?"

"That I never want to wash dishes again."

"Nothing else?"

"That's enough."

He took a drag on his cigarette. "It's better to earn a living with your mind, than your back."

They were among the words I would live by and why

I would always be by his side to help him start his own businesses.

"Wanna cuppa?" he asked.

"Sure, Dad."

He poured a cup of coffee for me and we sat, enjoying each other's company without saying anything more because just to be in each other's company was enough.

CHAPTER SIXTEEN

Coffee, Cigarettes and Sex

Coffee has always been part of my life: the smell, the sound of it percolating, and the warmth of the cup in both hands on a cold winter morning before school—but especially for the memories it brings of the late night cups and discussions I had with my father, the many cups I shared with Danny and Roy at our Sunday Brunches, and while waiting for Zev at his home.

Listening to the sound of my father's brew as it percolated musically and the aroma wafted up to my attic bedroom was almost like the chirping of birds in the morning for most people, but it was Brooklyn. Even the birds needed caffeine. I looked forward to the first cup in the morning with my father, if I could actually get myself out of bed in time to spend a few moments with him before he went to work and after he came up three times, imitated reveille, pulled the covers off me and sprinkled me with cold water. Then we would sit and talk as I put some milk and sugar in the brew and watched the spoon stand straight up in the center of the cup. More milk. Then college. Less milk. College full time and work 50 hours, six days a week. No milk. Straight caffeine. All seven years and four schools with time off for good behavior twice because it was all too much: too much education; too much work; too many divorces, remarriages, illnesses and adjustments to life. Thank God for work in Greenwich Village in the Sixties, the beautiful women in mini-skirts, the music that pulsated with every moment and shook the walls, the explosion of color and all the distractions from real life.

I finally gave up caffeine many years ago after I got married because my tolerance changed and it kept me awake at night when I actually wanted to sleep. It is a well-known fact that you can't live in New York City and sleep at the same time. You might miss something. Smoking, however, has never been part of my routine, though inhaling third party smoke was always second nature because my father and the second wife would smoke in the house, at restaurants, and in the car with the windows rolled up during the winter when we took a drive to enjoy the beauty of the Connecticut countryside.

By the time my wife and I were ready to go back home, I couldn't wait to get into my car. I went for the glove compartment, grabbed the bottle of Excedrin and swallowed a couple of tablets of more caffeine. But my head was still splitting open, and as soon as I got home I lay paralyzed on the couch until I fell asleep. Now I must monitor what I eat and drink to keep the sodium low, the oil virgin, and the bread at a minimum. Exercise, which I have been doing for many years, is still a must for body and mind, productivity at work and relaxation. The latest news: I'm back to regular coffee in the morning because it's good for health and longevity, along with a glass of red wine at dinner and some really good dark chocolate … in moderation, of course. And I'll never give up pizza. Kill me first.

• • •

Smoking, however, was always in the background of any conversation with my father that I pursued as I begged him to stop. But what was never really discussed then and isn't part of an open conversation now is the affect of the prostate treatment on sex. Impotence is written about as a side effect and doctors bring it up in passing, but there is no real public dialogue about it. It is quietly digested as a trade-off for treatment of prostate cancer because, let's face it, if you want to destroy the cancer, this is the side effect.

My father mentioned impotence once dismissively, but not using the actual word; so I listened, unsure whether to ask a question or make a comment, because he had been through so much. He was alive and I was thankful. I am alive and I am thankful. Whether I can have an erection or can ejaculate was not an issue important enough in my mind compared to eliminating the cancer, or at least stopping it from growing and spreading. That decision was not difficult for me to make. However, the thought of impotence can be devastating. Even if you open up to your wife, your girlfriend, family, friends or a support group, the result can't be changed. That point was made clear in the New York Times article and subsequent reports: Is the reliance on the PSA score and treatment for prostate cancer worth the side effects and problems?

When men approach the subject of sex, it becomes much more than a discussion about cancer; it is an issue of gender and culture, and the word "impotent" takes on many nuances. Sometimes it becomes a dismissive, humorous reference with self-conscious laughter on the part of the person making the insensitive remark: "Can you still do it?" But who wants to admit that he can't? Now we discover a lonely, invisible burden in which men are expected to live up to the image portrayed in TV and film to be always ready to perform. The response to "Can you still do it?" is simple: Don't ask. Don't tell. It didn't bother my father. I wouldn't let it bother me. Perhaps this is because prostate cancer is not identifiable. But, as we discussed in one workshop of breast cancer survivors, what was acceptable for men: baldness, natural, or otherwise, went unquestioned. It was a striking reminder, however, that a woman must be ill to be understood. Women don't become bald without a reason, and a wig becomes the temporary solution. Gender discrimination is part of our culture and society, and this double standard is not easily discussed because a woman who loses her hair causes a sense of shame. No one stares at a man.

CHAPTER SEVENTEEN

The Side Effects Have After Effects

The death of a loved one does not end when he or she dies. You don't go to sleep that night and wake up the next morning to find the world in place. Questions linger and remain unanswered; but who wants to bring up the disturbing complex issues of responsibilities and obligations to a person who is dying? How do you address these concerns with family and friends who are uncomfortable discussing them? Everyone, however, knows they are coming, and I knew I would have to tell my grandmother that my father died in a heartbreaking phone call that I dreaded making.

As soon as she heard my voice she started crying and wailing about her only son. There was nothing else I could say. Now my wife and I were faced with the one issue that could no longer be avoided, and there was no discussion or choice: We had to take care of my 88-year old grandmother.

I had begged my father to prepare me for the inevitable. I pleaded with him to provide me with the details and documents necessary to take care of my grandmother, but he insisted the second wife would do it. She had promised. She had given my father her word, and even though we both knew she would never keep her promise, he wanted to believe it; but as he reassured me time and again, he would not look me in the eye. Within a week after his death, my grandmother called to tell me that she had received a letter from the second wife's attorney cutting all ties, responsibilities and obligations. It was no longer her problem. But, and especially because I was the eldest of three sons, it was mine. Now I needed all the documents necessary to deal with my grandmother's affairs and continue her care. Who had that information? You know who.

The next step was to retrace all the work my father had been doing to keep my grandmother in her small studio apartment in an Art Deco building on Ocean Drive across from South Beach in Miami Beach, and I didn't have too much time to make decisions. The rent was rising because the landlord was trying to get all the elderly residents out in order to sell the building in anticipation of the Art Deco revival. Moving into a full care nursing home was way beyond my grandmother's means because she would live a lot longer than her finances would allow. So the obligation fell upon me. Well, not exactly. It fell upon my wife … with a thud. Ultimately, it would become her duty because as a woman she would have to bear much of the burden for caring for my grandmother. As we confronted the issues that would determine how we lived, it became clear that no one else was remotely interested in offering a helping hand: Cancer has side effects for the patient and after effects for the rest of us, and they last a very long time.

Was my grandmother, who had proved Darwin's theory of evolution and natural selection, about to make me another statistic? She had survived my grandfather, outlived my father and, as I was soon to learn, might bury me. The first day she entered our home in Connecticut, she laughed and said that our house was too small and her bedroom that we had labored over for a month to make perfect for her care was even smaller. And by the way, there's too much green everywhere. Welcome to lovely

Connecticut. She snickered, and I put my fist into a solid oak bedroom door. My broken knuckles and the inability to drive for the next month because I couldn't close my hand portended the future: Now my wife had to take care of my grandmother **and** me. The door didn't seem to notice, but I should have known it was coming.

• • •

From day one, the challenges grew intense. If my grandmother had had an education, she would have trampled everyone in sight and risen to the top of a major multinational corporation to become the first woman CEO. She took no prisoners, but she did take names. She counted birthday cards and holiday greetings from all the people who "loved" her and corresponded with her. In exchange, she sent a few dollars. She also had me read each and every card to her several times a week for my benefit at the beginning of our lives together. What an honor and privilege it was to be in her company and serve her. But she would break down in tears because it was so difficult for her to accept my father's death. She reminded me several times a day that he was her only "son," as if he was not my only father. I was a stranger about to enter an even stranger relationship and learn more about my father, my grandfather, and myself, than I ever thought I could know—and then I wanted to know more.

As I our lives together became more intimately entangled, I was encountering some very unusual aspects of my own personality in hers. It seemed as if certain of her character traits had skipped a generation, passed over my father, and transferred directly to me. I had always thought of myself as a completely independent person, but with each conversation my grandmother and I had, with each reaction to circumstance and attention to detail, I was learning that I had the same passion and tenacity that had driven her life. My father, however, usually calm and relaxed, knew when to stop and move out of the way of an unstoppable force. But she was relentless and unflappable and she drove him to distraction, as she did with my grandfather and now me.

I had to ask myself one question that would never be solved: How do you deal with a person who does not know when or even how to give up? Or one who never cedes control? Sometimes you have to observe the situation impartially and laugh. When my father and my youngest brother were visiting her in Miami one weekend, she called the police after they had gone to an early movie and didn't come back exactly on time to take her out to dinner. I also discovered that I had my grandfather's temper and intolerance, so as I got angrier at my grandmother's behavior, she continued to make remarks and snicker, infuriating me more. Then, as she did with my grandfather and father, she dealt the final blow, ignored me, and laughed.

CHAPTER EIGHTEEN

A Brush With Fate

Taking care of my grandmother was not only a reminder of my father's death, but of the stories we shared and the memories that were part of my DNA. My grandparents had lived in Atlantic City for many years before moving to Miami Beach and I loved my visits there. Listening to my grandfather's tales about his travels through Europe, Mexico South America, and Australia, as well as Japan, in his accented, but almost perfect English added exotic charm and my longing for more of his stories. Grandma Rosie was delighted to fill me in about all her problems adjusting to her new life in South America and how she had to learn Spanish and Portuguese to survive in Brazil, Argentina, and Uruguay. She did this quite well while she was taking care of my father as he was growing up because my grandfather was away so often. It was an exotic lifestyle that lasted for ten years.

Sometimes my grandfather and I took a ride on the rolling chairs along the Atlantic City boardwalk, or I went for a long stroll with my father. I was allowed to venture out on my own, and I stopped in at F.A.O. Schwartz amazed by all the life-size stuffed animals. I was mesmerized by the gravel-throated barkers who promised everyone a gift if they stayed just a moment longer and watched him chop up all kinds of vegetables with lightning speed. I sat in the back of storefront auction houses where gems and treasure boxes with undetermined contents were offered for a small sum that continued to grow. My cousin and I even sneaked into the burlesque a couple of times to watch middle-age strippers on stage and old men in the dark. What a thrill!

Grandma Rosie came to us with these memories and more. Grandpa was a chemist who traveled around the world and rarely came home, except when he was exhausted from sitting in airports and moving from one hotel suite to another. Staying away for long periods of time seemed to have something to do with the fact that on the few occasions when he did return to sleep in his own bed, my grandmother had given it to one of her sisters whom she seemed to invite over at exactly the same time, all the time, and he was forced out of the house and onto the tarmac again. But there was something else going on, and why two people from such opposite worlds ever got married was a complete mystery until I saw a picture of my grandmother as a young woman: She was stunning, but uneducated, and believed she deserved everything the world could offer. There was no doubt in her mind that she should be pampered. Then she met my grandfather, who had run away from home in Austria at the age of 16 because he didn't get along with his father. He traveled the world, received his education, and learned six languages, as he mastered his profession in the world of chemistry. He also had to evade the Nazis during his journeys in and out of Europe in order to bring his siblings and their families to America.

● ● ●

My grandfather did not have the same relationship with his father, and my father did not have the same relationship with my grandfather as he had with me. My father told me how much he resented my grandfather's absence during the time they were in South America and that he wouldn't speak to him for many years. It was only later in life that he understood why my grandfather was away for so long and so often, perhaps too late for him to completely reconcile with my grandfather. We, too, would learn why my grandfather could not stay home, as our time with Grandma Rosie continued, and endless day ran into endless night. But there were other stories, too.

On one of my grandfather's trips, as he was attempting to cross the border from Germany to France, he had to wait in line behind another man to present his papers. This was extremely dangerous because he could not identify himself as Jewish. Yet, he had to present some old, unreadable documents and try to talk his way to safe passage. My grandfather was also apprehensive because he had diamonds sewn into his pants cuffs and hidden in the seams of his jacket. As the German guard scrupulously examined a set of papers and questioned the man in front suspiciously, there was a sudden blackout. During that time, a vision of my grandfather's father came to him and told him that he need not worry because he would be allowed to pass safely. The lights came on and the man in front was gone. The guard adjusted his eyes, squinted at my grandfather, and waved him on. It was a story my father took some pleasure in telling, because my grandfather hadn't spoken to his father in many years since he had left Austria. His father was also dead by that time.

CHAPTER NINETEEN

An Indomitable Will of Steel and "The Girl"

Of course, I should have known what to expect before my wife and I went to Miami to get my grandmother ready to come up north. My grandmother was famous for being difficult and for ALWAYS getting her way, but our expectations were high and I had made a promise to my father. The house was prepared, we were thoroughly exhausted, and my grandmother seemed happy to leave her studio apartment and live with family. My wife boxed the relatively few belongings, including her clothing that fit into a few suitcases, and we were ready to go … shopping, because my grandmother wanted to pick up a few last minute things, as if she couldn't get them in Connecticut. So my wife stayed behind to prepare for the flight, and I left the beach for Collins Ave. and Lincoln Road, the center of the universe for everyone over 80. I went to flag down a taxi and before I got one foot off the curb, my grandmother, in her light blue cashmere sweater, light woolen beige coat with a silk scarf tied firmly around her head, was breaking the sound barrier. She did a marathon sprint on her fragile chicken legs to the stores leaving me in the whoosh behind her. By the time I found a taxi, she was halfway to our destination: the pharmacy. Pick up her medications? Not exactly.

"What do you want? I'll go get it and we'll go back home," I said helpfully, hopefully, and naively.

"I need some Tampons."

My body pulled to a dead halt in front of the double-eyebrow cosmetics. "What?"

Apparently, I was an idiot.

"Uh … You're 88. You need what?"

With one withering look she disintegrated me. Didn't hear me the first time? Do you know anything about women?

Then that commanding smirk that had defined her relationship with my grandfather and my father appeared, and I was compelled to acquiesce and surrender control. I compliantly approached a young woman who was working behind a counter and I whispered Grandma Rosie's request.

"Excuse me? Could you speak a little louder?" the clerk said, furrowing by her eyebrows in confusion: It's not that I can't hear you but did you just say what I think you said?

I muttered "Tampons" again under my breath.

"You need what?" she said and challenged me so the whole store could hear.

"Tampons."

"Tampons?" she asked me in what I could only hear as a broadcast voice at a stadium. "Tampons?" she said again in a normal voice that sounded like a cry for help. Unable to restrain herself from one more episode in the land of make-believe, she paused as the question mark hung in the air.

"I, uh ..."

"What kind do you usually buy?" she asked, grinning.

I shrank. "I think you'd better ask her," I mumbled, wallowing in humiliation and pointing to my grandmother.

"Who?" Oh, you've got to be kidding emanated

from her pores.

My throat went dry as I continued to shrivel.

"She's like 80," the young woman said.

"88, and I think you should talk to **her**," I begged, trying to hide my desire to flee that was seeping from every part of me. "**She**," I emphasized, "wants Tampons."

The young woman shook her head in disbelief and led the way imagining the story she would tell everyone else in the store after we left. "Mam, may I help you?"

Grandma Rosie just looked at her.

"You're uh … man … said you need Tampons?"

"Oh, God …" I could see the clerk's eyebrows above her head.

"You never know," my grandmother responded and ignored us.

Please don't make me pay for it, I repeated silently to myself like a chant.

"He'll pay for it," Grandma Rosie ordered: He'll also carry it for me.

Next, something simple: We were going shopping for shoes. Thank God, something simple. Shoes. How could that be a problem?

She wore AAA width to assist the chicken legs that

dug ruts into the ground when she wasn't moving forward. What could happen? And then it happened. She was in the store so fast I thought she had walked through the glass window. By my side one minute, gone the next. Little fingers of anxiety started to edge up the back of my neck as I tried to make myself casually invisible. I ducked from one aisle to the next, following her, as she scanned every single shoe that was displayed on top of a slanted shelf, hooked by the heel to a narrow strip of wood in the back to keep it in place. They thought. My grandmother marched with steadfast determination, touching the toe and flipping the heel up until the shoe was on the floor. Now I was on my knees, crawling military style as if I were carrying an automatic weapon, but gathering shoes in my arms and replacing them on the shelves anywhere they would fit, hoping no one would notice as people mostly older than 70 stopped what they were doing and pointed at me. Finally, I rose from my knees, a position I was getting used to, and was just about to pick her up and carry her to the exit, when she just walked out of the store. "Not my size."

• • •

Grandma Rosie never waivered from her resolve to

get her way, no matter how we tried to please or persuade her, a constant reminder of the "after affects" of dealing with terminal illness. My wife's home cooked food wasn't good enough. Grandma Rosie wanted to go to the diner. The coffee wasn't hot enough. It had to be scalding. My grandmother would rather eat out than have a healthy, home cooked lunch or dinner that my wife would spend hours preparing. And it was a major event when we did go out to eat because as soon as we entered the diner, her choice for elegant dining and gourmet food, she introduced me to the host and servers as if I had never been there before and she was a regular. She didn't pass a table or anyone waiting for a table who didn't need to know who Rose Meth was and who was by her side: her grandson and, as everyone else assumed so many years ago because my wife is Japanese, well to them "Oriental"— no, let me be more accurate—not white: Please allow me introduce you to her "personal aide," because Grandma Rosie's arm was looped through hers to keep steady. We had arrived at the pinnacle of life: The grandson, the grandmother, and the "girl." My wife was thrilled beyond words.

No sooner than the food came, Grandma Rosie went

for whatever was on my wife's plate and mine. No offer to order anything else she wanted could take the place of "sampling," as I had seen so many times at dinner with my grandfather and my father. My wife and I cut pieces from what we were eating and tried to put them on her plate. Not good enough. The battle raged on with my fork in one hand and my knife in the other. Grandma Rosie poked. I parried. She feinted. I fell for it, and she stabbed another French fry. I tried to protect myself, as my wife looked for another table, but Grandma Rosie moved with the speed and acuity of a master swordsman. She was in her territory and, as my grandfather did, other diners were fleeing. Unfortunately, we couldn't.

"More coffee!" she demanded. "You call this hot?" she sneered.

"More coffee," I requested meekly. "Please," I begged the waitress who smiled at this rare display of pure instinct for survival.

It was the serfs versus the warlord, and it was a humiliating defeat for us. As much as it infuriated my grandfather and my father, I could feel their smiles from above, as I shared their responsibility and mortality.

Taking care of another person is serious business,

especially an elderly person. It was her will against ours, and she was chipping away at mine, as she did with my father and grandfather—relentlessly and, of course, winning. When we bought her a beautiful cashmere sweater for her birthday, it wasn't the right color. She barely looked at me and dismissed it with a flick of her wrist. She didn't want pink. She wanted blue to match her eyes. When I explained that the store didn't have blue, but it was a very fine sweater, she told me to take it back. Several days a week, every week for the two years she spent with us, we had to take her to one doctor after another because she had accumulated so many problems during her many years alone.

In Miami Beach, the building was semi-independent and provided a cleaning staff. In our home, she once told me to get the "girl" to clean her room. Who? "The girl." My wife? My grandmother laughed, as if her innocent mistake had no meaning. But she was talking about my wife, the one person who was now devoting most of her waking moments to her, and who was now doing jumping jacks and stretching before she served dinner. When we took my grandmother to the ear doctor because she couldn't hear well, even with a new hearing aid, the doctor found pieces of cotton from a Q-Tip embedded in her auditory canal that were becoming fossilized. When her primary care physician told her told her not to breathe so he could check her heart, my grandmother was outraged. "Don't breathe?" she protested. "I gotta breathe!" The eye doctor. The diner. The cardiologist. The diner. The dermatologist. The diner. The diner. The diner. The nursing home. The cemetery. But who would go first?

CHAPTER TWENTY

Grandma Rosie's Revenge

It wasn't until we came back after teaching one night and smelled something burning that we realized we could not care for Grandma Rosie much longer. My wife ran to the kitchen where my grandmother had put a prepared dinner into the toaster oven, complete with its plastic packaging. We caught it just before the kitchen, and then the house, went up in flames. "I gotta eat!" my grandmother said in her defense. Yes, we do, too. We also have to live to eat. Or, as my father used to joke: "I eat to live. I don't live to eat." What goes around comes around, and now it was my turn, as my father and grandfather watched us from above, played pinochle and smoked. Our tour of duty turned out to be two years because, as Grandma Rosie became frailer, the demands of care became more intense, and she became more demanding. We had reached our limit. We couldn't handle her care, complaints, obstinacy, incontinence, and more visits to the doctor than I could count.

She also kept us up all night because she was constantly padding around with her walker, or dragging it behind her, and flushing the toilet every hour on the hour. So one night, I slipped downstairs quietly and watched as she walked from her bedroom to the kitchen to the bathroom and back, carrying her walker at times so she could get to her destination more quickly. She would stop in the bathroom, flush the toilet, and make the rounds again. She even looked in my direction as her instinct for survival told her that a predator was spying on her, and it spooked me.

The next morning, when I asked her what she was doing, she had no answer. When I asked her why she was flushing the toilet every hour, she looked at me like a child who had been caught being naughty. She needed 24 hour care, and we still had to teach, so we searched for an adequate local nursing home that didn't look like a scene out of One Flew Over The Cuckoo's Nest. It wasn't easy to find in those days. When I explained to her that we could no longer take care of her, she said: "I'm not going. I'll eat bread and water." Well, she was going, or we were going. We did what we could and it was wrecking us; but it had to be done and there was no one else who would take on the responsibility, not even to give us a weekend off. We were done.

The first night after she moved out, we slept; but I woke up occasionally listening for her, as if being awakened by the absence of activity or noise when a child is too quiet. I had not realized how attuned to her behavior we had become and how she had taken over our lives. We also had to catch up on several years of sleeplessness since my father's illness and death. Now we would be free, almost, until she died, which was not too long after her residency at the nursing home. The official record says she died of "Pulmonary Arrest." I know the truth. She continued to be in control until the last minute and refused to eat. If she had become a political dissident or fought for women's rights, or anyone else's rights in addition to her own, she would have changed the course of history. I made arrangements to have her remains cremated and my wife and I flew to Miami so she would be buried next to my grandfather, if he weren't on another flight out. That was the plan.

• • •

At La Guardia Airport we had to find long-term

parking, take the shuttle bus from the lot to the terminal, get on line to board the flight, and we were off. Plan A. By the time we found the entrance to the long-term parking lot after circling the airport several times, there wasn't a spot available within sight of the terminal, any terminal. So we parked way at the back, wherever that was, in another borough, and began unpacking, as we watched the bus waiting to take us to the terminals leave. It was hot, I was 30 pounds overweight and about to lose my mind as I attempted to jog to catch up to the bus, yelling at the driver to stop. There wasn't another bus in sight and we were running out of time. When a bus finally came and the driver graciously pointed to the designated spot where we could board, he was kind enough to allow us to hurry on, catch up, and wait as it continued to make half a dozen stops for other passengers. The flight to Miami was looking less and less probable. But we did arrive at the terminal with a little time to calm down, get ourselves together, put the trip in perspective, and … there was a bomb scare. Everyone was ordered to leave all suitcases and belongings and exit the building. More time passed. Finally, without explanation, the threat was over and we managed to actually get our tickets and secure our boarding passes with the ultimate goal of boarding the plane. With a great deal of relief, we checked our bags. I checked my sanity, and entered the plane. Oh, and … Champagne please. One more if you don't mind. Another would be nice.

We rented a car at the Miami airport, loaded the suitcases in the trunk and sat Grandma Rosie's ashes in the backseat with a seatbelt around her. About a half-hour into our journey I got a chill and I must have turned pale, because my wife asked me what was wrong. Grandma Rosie was sitting there, grinning and pointing a long bony finger at me and snarling as clearly as yesterday through the rearview mirror: "Heh, heh, heh …"

"Where are you going?" my wife asked as I got off the highway.

I pulled into a small shopping center, as my wife watched me suspiciously. I opened the rear driver's side door and ran my hand over the back seat. The box with her remains was still intact.

"Let's get some coffee and a bite to eat," I said and turned off the ignition.

Then I turned the ignition off again. I twisted the steering wheel, put my foot on the brake and tried to pull the key out of the steering post. But the key would not turn its full cycle and the ignition would not shut off. The engine, however, did. I think. I could hear it whirring, clicking and buzzing. We went into the coffee shop to get something for the rest of the half-hour trip, restart the engine and head for the cemetery. And then we heard the sirens. Smoke was billowing from the hood of the car and there were sparks.

Please, God, don't tell me! I ran to the car and struggled to open the doors. Naturally, they were locked because those were the days when you could leave the car running and still lock yourself out. "Heh, heh, heh …" Grandma Rosie was sitting in the back seat, staring through the window and pointing her bony finger at me. I had an extra key, unlocked the car and got the rear door open. I quickly removed her ashes and went around to the trunk. But that wouldn't open and sparks were shooting out causing a crowd to gather as flames burst from under the hood. A fireman yelled at me to get away from the car, but when he saw I wouldn't leave, he came rushing over.

"Get away from the car!" he yelled. "It can explode."

"I'm on my way to the cemetery," I replied.

"There are easier ways to go," he said with a perplexed expression and took the key, opened the trunk and handed me the suitcase.

I had the key in upside down.

Grandma Rosie turned to watch from the rear window.

At the cemetery, with 10 minutes until closing, the administrator in the office, who was also the owner, told me there wasn't enough time to bury her.

"What?"

She barely looked at me, but her dismissive smile stayed: Anything else?

"I just came from Connecticut and I've got my grandmother strapped in the back seat."

The fact that there had been a bomb scare, and my car blew up seemed not to impress her. Come back tomorrow. Oh, yeah? There is no way I'm going to sleep in the same hotel room with Grandma Rosie, dead or alive, ashes and spirit. I wouldn't leave the cemetery without granting her final place of rest. Period. Non-negotiable. So we were told where the plot was, given a map, and I drove to meet the attendant who would put this experience to rest. A half-hour later, about to jump out of my skin, I was back at the office. Where was the plot? I asked the locked door. No response. Another 15 minutes and we found a worker in a truck kind enough to take us to the plot. Even he couldn't read the map. But he did have a shovel.

I placed Grandma Rosie in the grave next to my grandfather, if he was still there, and it was over. There was also an inscription I had made on the stone in memory of my father: "Beloved mother of Benson and grandmother of David, Harold and Marc." She and my father were together again, if only in spirit, because my father was buried in Connecticut, waiting for the second wife behind a locked iron gate. Now we could leave. Well, I couldn't. I broke down in tears as my wife took a deep breath and rubbed my back.

CHAPTER TWENTY-ONE

The Love of Food, The Food of Love

Much is written about the role of food and nutrition in preventing cancer and the proper diet during and after treatment. Not much is mentioned about the emotional and psychological part food plays in relationships. Taking in and living with my grandmother after cancer had finally taken my father allowed me to see how generous another person can be in shouldering a responsibility that was not included in "until death due us part." My wife was devoted, patient and selfless. She had no idea how these qualities would be tested over and over again during our marriage, but she shared her love and spirit with my father and me, as well as everyone else in my family, and it added light to the day. She also added carrots.

My wife made a wide variety of delicious dishes, because that is one of the ways she and her family expressed their love: They took the time to show how much they cared about you by preparing food that reached directly to the heart. She spent hours in the kitchen creating a Japanese specialty or Italian recipe for my mother and the second husband when they came to visit, as well as for my father and the second wife whenever they came to our house, and they could smell the fragrance of her food before they got to the door. My wife extended herself in this way for other members of my immediate family during extreme hardships for years at a time, as well as for friends and acquaintances, because a gesture of love lasts forever. When you share food that is homemade in which the main ingredient is love, words are not necessary. Love and food speak their own language.

However, not all languages translate easily and immediately. My wife had left Tokyo, where we had met and I was still teaching, a year earlier than me for Santa Monica to work as an interpreter and translator. I moved to Los Angeles to be near her and she invited me to her apartment one night for dinner. That's a good way for a romance to blossom, as another old cliché goes: The way to a man's heart is through his stomach. Truer words could not be said in my case, and it was apparent that she had put a lot of thought into this dinner because she was making hamburgers. What a reward for a kid from Brooklyn. It was also a test from the first bite as I sank my teeth into it because she embedded it with ... Oh, please do not make this true ... Carrots! I had to eat a burger with carrots. Not even a cheeseburger. I did my best to seem appreciative, but what can I say? I'm from Brooklyn. I don't eat burgers with carrots. Nobody I knew would order a carrot burger. I have never even heard of a burger with carrots. Nobody in his right mind would put it on a menu. I want a cheeseburger and a bun sopping with fatty juices. Give me a grease burger, please, and a chocolate eggcream! But I ate it and I had to bite my lip as I told her how "special" it was. That I had never had **anything** like it before. I am still apologizing, because to verify when this happened, as I refreshed my memory to write this book, I asked her if this incident occurred in Tokyo. No, she told me, she wouldn't have a made a burger of any kind for me in Tokyo because she didn't love me that much. How much? Not as much as she could ever imagine at the time. And it was a German style hamburger steak, for your information. No bun. What did I know, anyway?

My wife is very creative, especially with food, and likes to experiment with new recipes. Well, maybe the recipes are not always new, and perhaps I'm just ignorant about certain foods, as she will look slightly away, raise her eyebrows and slowly lower her lids to attest. Shortly after I introduced her to my family, we went to Connecticut for dinner and she brought a cake that she had baked that afternoon. When we finished our dinner, she began serving this quite scrumptious looking chocolate cake and my father couldn't wait. It was chocolate and from his daughter-in-law to be. Perfect! Wonderful! He dug his fork in, took a taste and time stopped. His face contorted, because that's what strange food does to you. You don't think about grimacing. It just takes over your whole being. Your lip does something obscene, your nostrils flair disapprovingly, and your eyes twitch. Often you start crying and look for an immediate way to escape, usually under the table. Naively, he asked what kind of chocolate cake it was. Beginning to sense that my father, like me, was a rather basic guy when it came to "eating to live," she answered politely with surprise and thinly veiled embarrassment: Carrot cake.

"**We eat chocolate!**" a voice screamed in my head. "Who eats carrot cake in Brooklyn? Brooklyn! Do you even know where that is?" I never said a word.

My knees started to weaken. The chair began to wobble. Laughter bubbled up from somewhere around yesterday and I held my stomach to keep from folding over. Where could I go to hide? My father was nonplussed with embarrassment. What should he do? Please don't look at me I said with my eyes. He did. And thus started a slow, controlled smile that went around the table as each of us looked at one other, but not at my wife, and tried to hide an uncontrollable urge to burst into laughter. Yeah, that worked out well. It was a complete breakdown.

My father didn't want this lovely young woman who was to be my wife to leave for Japan directly from the house, so he beamed at such a special offer by her to become part of my family.

"Thank you, my daughter-in-law to be," he said graciously and lifted his fork.

But Ben Meth was who he was, and getting him to stab that cake again was another matter. He tried. There was some magnetic force pulling his arm back. I tried and broke into profound sweat. Carrots in hamburgers? We all looked at each other without saying a word. Carrots in cake? What next? Carrots in salad? Carrot juice? Who exactly was I living with? We forced ourselves to take another bite and it was spectacular. No apologies. Just embarrassed laughter. Food brings people together. Laughter makes you part of another person's life. Writing about it brings back these wonderful memories. Thank you. Thank you. Thank you to my wife and my father.

CHAPTER TWENTY-TWO

Duck Soup

No matter how difficult it was every day was a new day. That was my father's view of life. It is also mine. Dealing with prostate cancer has reinforced this awareness about my own health and future, because if you are not positive in your attitude from the time you wake up every morning, you cannot possibly succeed. No matter what you face, you must be productive and move forward. This is what I learned from my father when he confided in me something that no one else but mother had known: He never graduated from high school. When my grandfather decided to return to the United States, my father expected to finish his senior year of high school in Brazil and go on to college, but World War II had broken out and he joined the military. No advanced education for a young man who spoke three languages, had lived in four countries and had served in the American military in a few others, because when he came home, he got married, got a job, and "You came along," he used to say fondly. Now he had to support a family. This caused a gap that haunted him all of his adult life. Although he learned whatever job he had to do quickly and rose with lateral promotions, he was never allowed to rise high enough vertically without a college degree. He probably could have gone to night school, but he wanted to make money.

One night after dinner, I saw my father looking over some large books spread out on the living room floor. He was rehearsing a sales pitch for his newest attempt: He was going to sell encyclopedias door to door in the neighborhood. It lasted a little while without much success. Still searching for another opportunity, his friend, "Big" Al convinced him to buy into a "shooting" gallery in Coney Island where customers shot BB rifles at targets, usually inside the gallery, but the rifles were chained to the counter just in case. From Memorial Day to Labor Day for several years, he worked late into the night and went to his day job the next morning. Sometimes during the summer I went with him to Coney Island, and it was a thrill: The Steeplechase, the brass rings I collected on the Carousel, the distorted images I saw of myself in the mirrors of the Fun House. No visit was complete without a trip to Nathan's Famous for thin roast beef sandwiches dripping in juice, or hot clam broth that my father loved in Nathan's secret back room in winter. I was enthralled by the multitude of barkers, storefront food vendors, the throngs of people coming and going without direction, and the excitement of all the galleries and sideshows. My father introduced me to his odd collection of eccentric colleagues and I felt special as I was treated to free rides on the speeding Steeple Chase horses and zooming in and out of Bumper Cars. Most of all, I wanted to be with my father. Wherever he went, I wanted to go with him. Whatever he did, I wanted to do with him. And the feeling was mutual.

This was all before he lost his leg and had the blood of 32 people from his office coursing through his body to keep him alive. It makes you think. We take life for granted until there is a hint that it can be taken away. Often we do what we have to do, not what we are able to do. Even when something terrible happens and we promise to change our lives, we get over it and resume life as normal, because normal is what grounds us: the familiar keeps us going. My father kept looking for new ventures and trying to create new opportunities. It took a great deal of courage, but he finally made the decision to quit his job and challenge his profession on his own. It took an enormous amount of work, determination and perseverance, but he was able to establish his own consulting firm and become independent, giving seminars in international traffic and transportation around the country. My wife and I helped out when we could, but when my father could no longer walk I was there by his side for as long as he was able to conduct business. He didn't want to give up until the last minute and he continued his seminars, even during strong doses of radiation. I met him in the morning to help him get out of bed, get washed, get dressed, and into his wheelchair. He did everything, although he was in great pain, because he wanted to complete what he set out to do. He did not want to cancel and disappoint the men and women who were attending his conference. As a matter of fact, he wanted them to return to their offices and profession feeling that they had spent their time usefully and accomplished their own educational goals in their fields. At the end of the day, he went to his room to rest and I went into the whirlpool or sauna to relax. I met him for dinner, and I will never forget these times and others that we spent together.

Unfortunately, he couldn't pass on his business to any of his three sons, who had either studied something else or had no interest. Part of his legacy, however, remains in audio recordings I made of his seminars where he taught younger men and women and had me leaving the room occasionally to hide and howl with laughter at references that no one else understood. When he declared that something was as easy as "duck soup," the reaction went from "Huh?" To "What?" To "Oh … that's another one of Ben Meth's sayings." He issued certificates to the attendees at the end of the seminars and got a standing ovation. It was a small reward for someone who did not have a college education, or even a high school diploma, by people who had graduated from college or had Master's Degrees.

CHAPTER TWENTY-THREE

Allowed to Cry

As the intensity of radiation increased during my cancer treatment, I noticed a change in my body that I couldn't quite describe. My wife, very sensitive to my reactions and needs knew that there was something different occurring inside me. People later said that I seemed tired and worn out. When I went to see my doctors, I told them that I was heating up. They understood it theoretically because it was in the studies, brochures and pamphlets. It was to be expected. Predictably, it was making me rush to the bathroom, burning day and night, and keeping me sleepless. What else is new?

It was nothing close to the frightening and wrenching side effects of what my father suffered, or what many, many other people must endure from different types of cancer. Words are not adequate here, but neither is silence. As uncomfortable as I felt, I knew I was being spared. I also knew the side effects were supposed to wind down after 4-6 weeks, as the nuclear half-life of the seeds ate away at itself for 67 days. Well, let's say a good four months for the side effects to simmer down, and six months for most of them to disappear, though a solid night of sleep is not a guarantee; nor is a normal sexual life. You have to give up something, but you must retain your dignity.

How you feel about yourself is paramount to recovery and good health. I continued work on the play I was writing and, fortunately, I was only a short drive from the university and theater where the cast had no idea I had started cancer treatment. Writing and working with the students was invigorating, even if I was tired. They must have thought it was unusual, but I was at every rehearsal with the director, whom I didn't tell that I had prostate cancer until about 15 drafts later when we were close to opening night. Being with the director and cast during the rehearsals gave me a sense of purpose, instead of sitting at home in front of the TV making an effort to get my mind off myself. Sometimes I came home late at night and did immediate rewrites while they were still fresh in my mind. I would try to sleep, but 15-20 minute increments seemed to be my limit and not really what anyone could call sleep. So I looked over what I had written and wrote some more. I usually had changes or a new draft that morning. When I was finally done with the play, I had brought to life characters and a story for other people to perform and see on stage. It was important in regaining my health because I had not lost focus and knew that I would recover. Instead of going from nothing to zero, I went from a blank page to a full stage. The imagination is very special. It is a creation. Even if you have never made the effort to write or stretched your imagination to its limits before, everyone has this ability. We are all creative and talented in some way.

I have proposed writing programs and workshops at all the local hospitals in the county where I live, and even the hospital where I was treated with the same result: no one was interested. Not even at some of the cancer care centers. There were support groups, art and music therapy classes, social workers and psychologists, many people with good intentions, but there was also a profound disconnect between patient and professionals when it came to expressing experiences and thoughts in writing. If I received a response, it was politely dismissive with no further explanation. Was it money? It never even came up for discussion. Was it a lack of interest? That's one likely conclusion, but how is it possible? Cancer is not just a physical disease. It cannot be treated separately from the patient and the family, or from its emotional and psychological impact on everyone concerned.

Much has changed in the treatment of cancer since my father's death. Not much has changed in our inability to communicate about this devastating disease. The least communication takes place between doctor and patient because we don't speak the same language. The doctors talk statistics and clinical facts, procedures and medications; the patient is guarded in fear of the unknown and doesn't know what questions to ask. When my father was being eaten alive by radiation and chemotherapy, even though he accepted it, I couldn't. I called his doctor and begged him to do more to relieve his pain, to enable him to eat. The doctor said there was nothing he could do. What? If **you** can't do anything, who can? Then the doctor broke down in tears on the other end of the phone.

As much as cancer is about treatment, it is very much

about communication; and medical professionals need to learn how to deal with their patients on a different level. When my father was under the care of a different doctor at a different facility, this doctor didn't always show up for appointments or return phone calls. I have been fortunate to have very caring and sensitive medical professionals who answered my questions and addressed my concerns as best they could; however, they still did not have a true understanding about what I was going through because that they had not been through the same experience personally.

How do we make this experience personal? Patients must write the script for their health and wellbeing, not the medical professionals. The narrative has to unfold by family and friends so that the medical professionals can hear what is never said. Doctors, nurses and other caretakers can bear witness or participate. They can also write their own feelings and thoughts for the patients to hear. They should be allowed to cry, too. However, the gap must be closed for true healing, even if the patient cannot always be cured. This is what keeping a journal or writing from a personal point of view can do.

CHAPTER TWENTY-FOUR

Performing Cancer

Sometimes you need to hear your thoughts and words out loud. Years after my father's death, I saw the play, WIT, written by Margaret Edson about an English professor who was dying from ovarian cancer. It was a beautifully written, engrossing drama with a good sense of humor, but I had no idea how powerful the play was until the end. The audience was leaving and the seats were being vacated, but I couldn't get up. I couldn't move. I put my head in my hands and began to sob uncontrollably. Slowly and without particular notice, the play had gone directly to my heart, and until the final curtain I was unaware of how much of my father's illness and death were still with me. The play had opened me up to events that had shaped my life and influenced my future because, even though the person you love may be gone, the memories and emotions never die. And you cannot know how what you write will affect someone else.

Journals. Dramatic narratives. Humorous stories. A play to be read out loud or staged. These reminiscences and journeys are not just therapy for the person writing them. They are an invitation to other people to share part of your life. This has been my experience in making my work public when members of the audience who have seen one of my plays come up to me and ask how I could know about some of the experiences they had and seemed to share with them. Of course, I didn't know.

I did, however, create one opportunity with the support of a nationally known, local center for survivors of cancer. I held a short series of writing workshops for cancer survivors that were very special successes. We had ten participants in each one, with some people who came to more than one. They included many professional women, at least one medical doctor, educators and, as we were to learn later, a participant who had suffered physical abuse. Although the participants didn't know what to expect, after brief introductions and my instructions about how the workshop was planned, participants began to relax. I discussed my background and relationship to cancer and then people who were at first hesitant to attend and then reluctant to write, began writing almost immediately.

It soon became clear that the workshop filled a need for personal expression of feelings, thoughts and memories that, although they were intimate, needed the support and comfort of other participants in the center's very warm and caring atmosphere. This was significant because writing should be a way to free yourself through exploration and self-discovery to come to terms with who you are. In other words, as I explained to the participants: Whatever you write is fine: a letter you may never send; a word, a phrase, an outline; a poem, a story, a conversation that you would like to have, but can't; a schism that was created and went unresolved, but which you can resolve on paper instead of going over it again and again when you close your eyes at night to go to sleep. The participants were free to ask me questions or seek direction about how to structure what they wanted to say into the form most appropriate for expression.

As participants went more deeply into their writing, a natural flow and beauty emerged, and the writers began to discover their own voices. This was revealed through one writer who said she had come across her mother's memoirs ten years after she died of breast cancer and wondered if she could respond to them on paper.

Everyone agreed it was a wonderful idea. The medical doctor expressed her disappointment about how she could only refer to patients as numbers and that she was accountable for every extra minute spent to get to know and comfort someone. But it must not prevent her from moving on to the next patient. That, she said, was not why she had become a physician.

One of the most dramatic moments occurred about thirty minutes into the first session when I left the room to get some coffee. As I was returning, one of the participants was leaving. I thought it was a momentary trip to the restroom, but she looked unhappy and I asked her if everything was okay. She said, "no." She confided to me that everyone was writing and she could not put a word on paper. When I asked what was preventing her, she replied that writing brought back too many terrible memories and it was painful. She opened up to describe some of those memories that she didn't want to discuss, in particular that she had been attacked. Her fear and frustration were overwhelming and her eyes became moist. I asked if she wouldn't mind returning and writing what she had told me, even if it was just a word here and there. It didn't have to be in sentences, but thoughts, ideas, or emotions as she expressed them to me; and she didn't have to show it to anyone. She went back to her seat and by the end of the session had two pages. She also joined the next session and wrote freely in outline form which, when she read it to the workshop, had the flow of a poem.

Another participant began crying as she wrote and, when she was done, insisted on reading it to the group because to write it was to free herself of the emotional constraints that the memories imposed. To read it out loud to the other writers was to make it real. As a result, many of the participants thanked her and those who shared their feelings and commented how touching their writing was. They also said that other members had expressed thoughts and emotions that they were unable to put into words, or said it more beautifully. Participants praised each other's courage. These writing workshops became part of our lives and memorable for all of us.

• • •

Being able to make your feelings known helps other people understand that they are not alone. When my father entered his first care center, a hospice, I gave him a blank journal and asked him to write down his thoughts for me to keep. After he died, the second wife sheepishly handed it back to me. It was blank, except for an inscription on the front page. It was dedicated to her, telling her how much he loved her. In spite of how unimaginably abusive she was to him, he still wanted her to know that he loved her and, by implication, that he forgave her. His heart was always open and full of love, and he taught us all a lesson even after his death. So I gave my father's last written words to her.

We need more than memories to carry on the spirit. Memories fade, but words live forever. How you convey your thoughts changes other people's lives because it can help them understand themselves. This is true for medical professionals, social workers and care providers, as well as the patients and their families because the healing process is personal, not just by appointment. To participate as an equal, however, means you must open your heart and bare your feelings.

CHAPTER TWENTY-FIVE

The Cancer Culture Conflicts

In American society, revealing your inner thoughts and emotions means admitting that you are vulnerable, and it goes against everything we are taught from the time we are children. It is especially true now, because we live in a time where communication is almost impossible to escape: phone calls, text messages, email, tweets, location identification and so much more. It is just as easy to ignore someone; and it seems more offensive now, since we expect an immediate response. In the past, when a hand written letter or card was received, it was greeted with joy, held to the heart, and preserved forever to read over and over. Now it is rare to receive one. Expressing feelings personally is washed away in digital communication, cute cards graphically illustrated or animated by a third party that you can't hold, and masses of information that you really don't need. Research online is taking the place of personal consultation because very few people have the time or care to devote the time to spend with another person; but if they must, at a price. Nothing is personal. Privacy is lost. You are who everyone thinks you are: It says so online, in surveys, ratings, scores and statistics, in addition to medical and credit reports. So, to admit to another person that you have cancer, or to confide that you are afraid, is to ask them to listen and understand, to request their personal time to share your life. In a world that is more burdensome than ever, who wants to sign on to someone else's problems?

As a result, too many people are afraid to communicate and they keep their concerns to themselves. When you bring your problems to a doctor, you are allotted a very limited amount of time and then you are rushed out for the next person in line. But you leave feeling cheated and angry. I feel cheated by doctors who keep looking at the clock or their watch, and lean toward the door when my 10 or 15 minutes are up. But the bill for $100.00 or more is already in the mail, if you are not required to pay up front and then told to find another medical group if you are unhappy with their policy. I leave the office angry when the doctor sends in an assistant who asks for my medical information a second time and then enters it on another patient's computer records, or asks me how my blood pressure is instead of taking it. I was incensed when I had to get dressed and leave the examination room after a half-hour to remind an incompetent, former urologist that I was in excruciating pain with a blood clot in my urinary tract from the TURP, because no one in the office remembered I was the first patient there at 8AM. As patients, we are supposed to accept what we are given and assume the medical professionals know what they are doing, even when they are distracted, unprofessional, or given incentives by insurance and pharmaceutical companies to promote a product or reduce costs.

How does this all reflect on cancer? It is the mindset of the medical profession: First is time. Next is money. Treatment follows, and, too often, the patient is last. Therefore, you must find exactly the right doctors who are skilled and compassionate, and whose primary goal is not rolling patients in and out of their medical group, but treating them as human beings. All of these considerations and decisions immediately begin to take a toll on the patient and family, and it is a great emotional drain. We are not just confronting our own personal battle, but we are squarely in the middle of the Cancer Culture Conflicts. The front lines dictate how we speak about ourselves, because we must carry our stress in silence: Don't reveal too much. Don't speak too soon. Once the information is out, who knows where it will go or how it will be used? I applied for a summer teaching position one time and the online form required my Social Security number with permission to access my credit history and medical records. I called up the head office and asked why they needed more information than is necessary to get a mortgage. They assured me that they would never use or abuse this personal data. Then don't require it. Then don't apply.

I have not been afraid or shy over the years to discuss how my wife and I dealt with my father's illnesses, and it gave comfort to some people to know that they were not the only ones going through such trials. Once, when I responded to a stranger's request online for advice on how to deal with a terminally ill parent, I got many responses thanking me for sharing my experience with them. Now that I have had and been cured of prostate cancer, I have found sharing what I was going through is beneficial to everyone interested in the conversation, except to the dozens of administrators of patient support programs at hospitals to whom I submitted proposals for writing workshops. What is missing here? Should patients, family and friends stay silent? I believe it is part of our culture to bury our troubles, rather than expose ourselves. Do you want your employer to know? Will you be able to remain at your job? Can you be let go? If you are fired, what is next and how much will it cost you to defend your rights? What about your out-of-pocket medical expenses, or the expenses the insurance provider won't accept? It goes right back to the doctors and insurance corporations and their vicious cycle of financial abuse by overcharging, underpaying and, finally, handing over the bills to the patient.

You may confide in your friends, but how much do they really want to know? My friends showed concern and shared their experiences, sometimes revealing problems that they had not mentioned before. I have been lucky to have best friends from the time I was growing up. They listened, they shared, and we helped each other. Your family will know by necessity, but soon it becomes their problem and, depending on how they deal with it, you, the patient, could actually become less important than the person "worrying" about you. Family members become a burden because someone may want to assume your pain and suffering. When they can't, they create their own. It's a serious issue because the patient has a double onus: his or her own illness and the suffering caused for the people he or she loves most. Often, people begin to express their concern with darkness in their eyes and the tone of their voice drops into depression that hurts the person who has been diagnosed with cancer or is undergoing treatment. An example of this attitude was reinforced in one workshop in which a breast cancer survivor described the many times people would say something inappropriate or insensitive. The only way she could deal with it without confronting the speaker and saying how awful it made her feel was to write the remarks down in a list and enclose them in her journal. Out of her heart and onto the page. Her experience encouraged the other members of the workshop to make entries in their journals and open up to discuss their own experiences.

• • •

As individuals, we have to share responsibility. But what happens when someone doesn't do his or her share, or avoids the situation? Worse, he or she suddenly appears and offers an unsolicited opinion without understanding the issues thoroughly. Consider what happens when one person assumes complete authority, and that authority is misguided, misinformed, or absolutely wrong. What if there is money involved? Everybody has his fingers in places they do not belong. When my father died, I knew that I had to take over the care of my grandmother; but life would have been much easier if, as a family, we were able to communicate and my father had written out the details of each person's obligations and responsibilities. Instead, it caused a great deal of confusion, anxiety and work, because no one besides my wife and I would take care of my grandmother. My wife could have refused. Instead, she assumed responsibility and our marriage survived. How fortunate I am to have married such a very special woman.

CHAPTER TWENTY-SIX

So Many Years Later

It is the American way to separate the human being into body parts. Each doctor looks at only what concerns him. More than one doctor means more than one diagnosis, more than one medication, and they may all conflict because no one sees the patient: they only look at the condition and only investigate the problem. Like an automobile, they service the part that needs repair. Come back if another part breaks down. Unlike an automobile, the cure for the person has side effects and the side effects have after effects. We become numbers and letters on charts, colors on a diagram, codes on a computer screen. We are data. But when no one asks how much I have slept, or if I have slept at all, I know that I have lost my identity as a person. Illnesses need to be treated. A person needs sleep. A person needs to eat. We need to enjoy what we eat. We need to talk and laugh and appreciate life. We remember and cherish good memories. The medical profession does not allow for this, but doctors need to see us as more than removing or replacing a part; they must accept us as people rather than the next appointment of the day.

We need to share our lives and experiences and support each other, not just offer care and express sympathy. That means exposing our vulnerabilities. Comedians do it by laughing at themselves and us in public. Laughter allows an emotional release that presents a look back at events that may have been terrifying or tragic at the time, but now seem unbelievable, and you wonder how you did it. Personal narratives, journals, all forms of writing allow the writer to take a situation that might have been intolerable when it occurred and purge it. It gives you permission to say all the things you wanted to say, but didn't or couldn't. It is an escape from the past so that the burden does not pursue you into the future. Sometimes what you write comes out naturally in a journal, as it did during the extreme difficulties of my father's illness; or it requires time to discover the right medium and words that best suit what you have to say. I found this to be true in a 10-minute dramatic play I wrote about the funeral after my father's death. I, too, wondered if I was alone in the way cancer affected my family and my life, because the death of a loved one does not end when he or she dies. The effects linger, but they should not take over.

• • •

Although I have survived the same disease that took my father, it took me over thirty years to write about my father's funeral. Even though so much time has gone by and it is easier to relive those moments from the distant future, I wonder how I dealt with certain experiences as I re-read my notes and letters.

The day that had come for the beginning of closure seems like yesterday. The final process for him to say good-bye to his family, friends and colleagues was here for us to pay our respects. My wife and I arrived early at the synagogue in the neighboring area of Southbury, CT where my father and the second wife lived, and my two brothers came soon afterwards. But no one was there to greet us. We waited in the lobby for thirty minutes as the Rabbi passed by several times without even looking in our direction. I went up to him as he hurried away from us and I identified myself, but he didn't acknowledge me or say a word. The second wife had set up the arrangements and it was clear that a line had been drawn from a single moment in the hospice when she declared that she didn't want to lose my wife and me after my father died because we were the "best thing" to come out of their marriage. We never spoke to her again.

She had infected the Rabbi and now he wouldn't grant us even the most basic courtesy or respect in our time of grief and closure, so we went into the synagogue and sat in the front row alone. A short time later, the Rabbi sent someone to ask us to come into a room to greet mourners and well-wishers with the second wife and her son because it would "look" better. I guess he did know who we were. I refused. So did my wife and my brothers. As people arrived, they paid their respects in the reception room and then came to Benson Meth's three sons, his flesh and blood, to pay their respects.

The Rabbi made a feeble eulogy and demonstrated that he didn't know my father or anything about him; but it was easy for me to speak deeply from my heart about the man whom I loved and was my best friend. The woman who told me about the "things" that took a long time and my father's "legacy" came up to me later and said she was sorry. I didn't look at her and walked on. At the end of the service, I left with my wife, my brothers, and my friend Danny and his wife to gather for a late lunch in my father's memory. I had no way to know that this last rite would last forever.

I called the Rabbi two days after the funeral because I hadn't heard about the plans for my father's burial, and he seemed preoccupied. I was interrupting him.

"We already …" he began, and caught himself.

"You what?" I raised my voice over the thumping of my heart, rose from my chair and started to pace.

"You buried my father without telling me?"

"When is the last time you called me?" he demanded arrogantly.

"Call you? Why would I call you? You wouldn't even acknowledge us after I introduced myself."

"Your mother is a member of my congregation," he said quickly. "I am responsible to her."

I was beyond livid. "She's not my mother, and my father was also a member of your congregation. What is your responsibility to him and his sons?"

He didn't know what to say, but he wasn't at a loss for words. "Listen …" he began presumptuously. It was clear. I didn't matter. My brothers didn't matter. Ben

Meth's sons didn't matter.

"What? What do you want to say to me about denying a man's sons their right to be at his burial? How do you justify denying us closure?"

"Listen, I don't have to …" he added, as I slammed the phone down and my fingers rolled into a knot that would not unfurl for many years.

CHAPTER TWENTY-SEVEN

Cancer as a Mutual Friend

In those years after my wife and I moved to Connecticut to take care of my grandmother and she took her place in the family history, we moved to another home where there was more open space and, as a result, more stories. This is when my neighbor and I got to know each other and immediately reduced our relationship to "got to know **of** each other" because it was over within days of our first encounter.

This estrangement began shortly after he called me to say that he was going to mow the wild wooded area that we shared in back of our houses to make space for his son to play soccer. This was his basic introduction, his rite of initiation. He went on to describe how he was planning to remove the bushes in the back that (by the way) helped prevent flooding from a brook that we also shared. In addition, I was downstream from the dam that he had built and controlled and went directly into my basement during storms because he never forewarned us that he was going to open the flood gates in order to prevent **his** property from being flooded.

When I said that I didn't think his proposal was a good idea because it would eliminate the little flood protection we had, he replied with an attitude that he was well known for in our small town. He was very calm and polite, and, as usual, explicitly informative: "I didn't ask you what you thought. I was telling you what I was going to do." That created the animus that would last for three decades. Yet, my neighbor, whose name I never uttered when words passed between us on a rare occasion, was a very talented, well-educated, stubborn man who could work magic with a backhoe when he wasn't tearing apart the town attorney with his bare hands and a quill pen. All alone, he built an addition to his house with calibrated clay roof tiles that he also designed. He drew up the blueprints, exceeded the code for wiring his house, hammered in every nail, screwed in every bolt, and raised extremely heavy lumber and tiles that would normally require a skilled team of men and a supervisor at a premium. He was older, but trim and physically fit from all of his endeavors and didn't lose a beat when it came to challenging the town.

He also built a beautiful wall between our properties with all the stones and small boulders that lined the brook, as he flattened out the embankment by traveling back and forth over it in his backhoe. When I pointed out the flooding in my basement, he implied that it was my problem and, by the way, the stones were not my property. He knew every rule, regulation, and code of our small town of 25,000 people and fought incessantly with everyone in authority and those who were not. Although most of the residents had formed very strong opinions about him, a few recognized his willingness to fight for what he believed, and no one wanted to take him on personally. All I wanted was not to be flooded or have my vision blocked when he parked his vintage Jeep on the sidewalk within the laser beam parameters of responsibility that made it difficult to measure and accuse him of any type of violation by the naked eye. The police did not want to issue a ticket, because he fought his own battles in court and forced the town to pay an attorney. And he never lost. At least, that's what everyone thought until he lost to me. It seemed to be a badge of honor when the police wrote this particular ticket for blocking a part of the street that impaired my vision of oncoming traffic. However, as accurate as my neighbor was, the judge didn't give in and sustained the $25.00 fine. That truly upset him.

As he did things on his property that defied common courtesy, he went to the edge of the rules and regulations established by the town, the state, and the federal government, and nothing could deter him—no one could over-rule him or enforce laws against him except for that one time. He was just to smart and his research was meticulous. We never spoke, but I did spook him a couple of times when I caught him flattening out the stream with his backhoe or pushing all of the weeds and overgrowth on his side of the brook to the property line so it would wash down onto my side and I would have to dredge it and remove it. It was, however, the age of digital cameras and I photographed it. I photographed him doing it. That really upset him, but even with such evidence, the town was afraid to confront him. He was like the massive concrete wall he had built in front of his house to the consternation of everyone who passed by and made a comment about the condition of his property. He was unmovable.

Until one day during Christmas when my wife asked me to walk over his house and deliver some chocolate chip cookies. She had become yard friends with my neighbor and his wife in polite conversations in back of our houses by the brook, and had been bringing them baked goods for a few years. This time it was my turn to extend the courtesy and offer of friendship. I, however, would not consider it. So she went to our neighbor's house and left the neatly wrapped, festive package on the doorknob when no one seemed to be at home. About a half-hour later, there was a knock on the door, and there he was. Please don't tell me, I thought, that he is going to return the cookies. No, that was not his intention. As he stood outside in some rather nasty, cold weather with icy rain beating down on his face, he made himself clear immediately: "I came over to say thank you." I was stunned.

"Please come in," my wife said over my shoulder.

I have tried to convince her to this day that I was planning to invite him in, rather than let him soak in the icy rain, but she still does not believe it.

So, this man, a few years older than me and with many years of animosity built layer upon layer that became impenetrable, entered my house. I took his coat and there he was, in my living room, sitting in my favorite armchair, feeling at home. How could this be? My wife asked him if he would like a cup of tea, and he graciously accepted. Then she asked him what kind of tea he would like and gave him a choice of at least a dozen different kinds, including several from Japan. Where could he get that?

As we sat together over tea and some other baked goods that my wife had made for the holidays, this man for whom the word "dislike" was a very mild understatement, was funny, quite charming, and self-deprecating. He had a slightly dark sense of humor, and that appealed to me immediately. He was also a very good storyteller. I tried not to let the words escape from my lips, but I couldn't ignore the feeling that was taking over: This is a guy I could like. We settled into more familiar conversation as if we were long time friends, and I mentioned that I had recently recovered from prostate cancer. He revealed that he just had been diagnosed with lymphoma and he was going into New York to begin treatment. The tea, by the way, was really nice. Where could he get it? My fondness for him kept growing and I couldn't help wonder what we had been missing all these years as we sat in front of the fireplace.

The weather warmed up and we saw each other occasionally after our brief Christmas introduction. He began repairing a fence that he put up between our properties many years ago and he was cordial, but still with a hint of defensiveness, even though I no longer posed a threat. My wife became more friendly with his wife, and he seemed to like that, perhaps because he felt it would be nice for her to have a friendly neighbor right next door when cancer finally overpowered him. That day came and many people in the town attended his memorial service. I, the person who never wanted to acknowledge him and went out of my way to avoid him, spoke about our relationship and said something that I have never said about anyone else except my father. My neighbor, a man who had alienated me from the first time we met, had taught me something very valuable: In spite of his character and temperament, we both ignored a relationship that could have developed into a deeper friendship. I should have been a more gracious person and overlooked his defensive attitude and shortcomings. I should have made an offer of friendship. I could have taken the lead, and I am sorry that I didn't. But I thank you for this very important lesson.

CHAPTER TWENTY-EIGHT

The Higher Education of Cancer

Not long after my short friendship with my neighbor, another friend who has a small family restaurant and makes the most delicious Italian food and pizza seemed at a loss for words after he asked how I was doing. I told him that my recovery for prostate cancer was going very well and he paused. A moment later he told me that his oldest daughter, a senior in high school, had just been diagnosed with thyroid cancer. She was going to begin treatment in a couple of weeks, and he took a moment to reflect on just how his family life had changed. Speaking out loud to himself, he wondered how she was going to do the intensive amount of work required by the college application process and meet all the deadlines while she was being treated for cancer? What if things didn't work out? No, of course they would work out. But … What if …?

Thyroid cancer. His daughter was 17, an excellent student, an athlete, and now a patient whose future had taken an unimaginable turn for her whole family. It was, he later told me, the worst three months of his life. I was encouraging, but when a child is diagnosed with cancer, encouragement is a sliver of dim light that seems to fade with each thought. The best I could do was to offer to help his daughter prepare for her college applications whenever she felt she was able to begin, for as long as she had the desire, energy, and determination because, as her father and I agreed: There was no doubt—she would recover.

From the moment I met her for the first time at the beginning of her final year of high school and after her treatment had begun, two words came to mind: strength and determination. From the way she walked, to her expression, no illness, no matter how serious it was, was going to defeat her. The energy and self-assurance that emanated from this young woman was clearly a statement: she would accept no obstacle in the way of attending college, and it gave her parents confidence. She would not only get well, but she would thrive. This is what her parents needed and what sustained them along with the support of her two younger sisters and brother.

As this lovely high school senior approached the table where I was sitting in a local café, she seemed to be making a fashion statement. Much different from what young women usually where these days, she was wearing a scarf. As she wrote in her essay, she needed to cover a three-inch incision that defined a personal battle she would have to overcome, and one that transformed her from a teenager to a woman when she returned from summer camp and saw her mother on the front porch with her head in her hands, crying. It was also as she says in her essay, that her mother dropped the "C-Bomb" on her and she shortly thereafter became Case #18397227. Cancer was no longer about other people.

She recounted the poking, probing, and prodding before and during hours of surgery. When she awoke from the haze of anesthesia and realized that she was still alive, she took a stroll in the hospital hall for a few minutes with her parents. A little baby was in another room connected to tubes and cables as the world beyond monitored her life and frightened her parents. But what could they do? These 300 seconds, she wrote, changed her life.

This college student is a force of inspiration through the power and beauty of her words, and I feel privileged to have worked with such a positive young woman whose strength of spirit could empower others. Passing on the craft of writing to nurture others is what teaching is about. Surviving cancer is indeed a shared experience. Working with young people to instill hope is how we all survive.

The Unclenched Fist

The years since my father lost his leg, his ability to conquer his first most serious battle with illness and survive, has stayed with me in many different ways. His power to remain positive and maintain a heartfelt sense of humor has always been part of my life. Yet, I still find myself changing because of the unexpected bonds that cancer creates between friends, acquaintances and strangers. Writing and speaking about my own experiences with cancer and sharing them help to heal beyond professional medical treatment. It actually goes far beyond that. The simple process of telling a story breaks down the psychological, emotional and physical walls to create the support that we all need and give us hope that love is never far away.

Sometimes I feel my father's gentle touch on my shoulder. Occasionally he greets me in a dream as he walks naturally without a limp and gives me a warm hug and a kiss.

"David, my son …" he whispers over my shoulder.

He is no longer in some dark, distant place that I can't identify, or where I cannot reach him. His smile is bright and there is light in his eyes.

We can't right all wrongs or change the past. We can't cure all diseases or be sure about what is coming down the street or waiting for us just off the curb. Words, however, last forever and certain offenses need time to fade from memory or generate a laugh.

We may also write another ending and create a new beginning, one that gives peace of mind and relieves the heart. I am very fortunate. I am cancer free, fit in body and mind, and although closure took a very long time, I have never been alone because my wife has been by my side and my father's spirit has always been with me.

My father did not pass away.

He passed on.

He passed on his sense of fairness, love, and inspiration to all who knew him.

I do not know when I will meet him next, but I am sure I will.

Thank you for allowing me to share my life and

experiences with you so together we may greet every day as a gift.

About the Author:

David L. Meth is a novelist and award-winning playwright who has been produced nationally and internationally. His first novel, **A HINT OF LIGHT**, received 5 stars on Amazon and 5 stars in South Korea where it has been translated and published in Korean.

A HINT OF LIGHT is the story of Byung-suk, a black-Korean Amerasian boy orphaned to the streets of Seoul who must make his way through the gutters and back alleys of the marketplace, in and out of whorehouses and hotels, and protect Miya, a young, half-white Korean girl who is mute. Trapped in their own skins because of their color, these children are foreigners in their own land with no identity and no escape. **A HINT OF LIGHT** is a dramatic view of the streets through the eyes of its inhabitants and exposes the underbelly of racism that permeates Asian and American societies. Yet these children never lose hope or give up on their dreams as they discover their talent for languages and take advantage of adversity to turn it into good fortune in their search of their fathers. The author spent three years on research, including a year in Korea and a year in Japan, and interviewed many of these children and people who cared for them.

Much more is on his website: DavidMeth.com

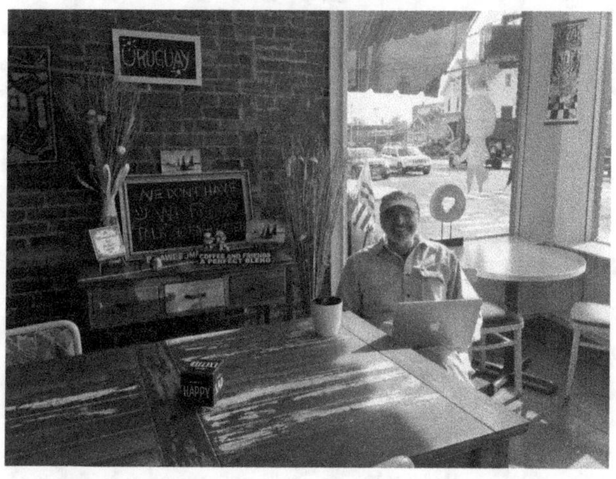

www.ingramcontent.com/pod-product-compliance
Lightning Source LLC
Chambersburg PA
CBHW070831250726
48662CB00003B/1164